Pocket Exan
Surgery

C000179080

Pocket Examiner in
Surgery

Second edition

John Northover MS FRCS
Consultant Surgeon, St Mark's Hospital, London

Tom Treasure MD MS FRCS
Professor of Cardiothoracic Surgery, St George's Hospital, London

David Melville MA DM FRCS
Consultant General Surgeon, North Middlesex Hospital, London

With contributions from:

Matthew Fletcher MS FRCS
Consultant Urologist, Brighton

John Dixon MCh FRCS
Consultant Orthopaedic Surgeon, Winford Orthopaedic Hospital, Bristol

Michael Bridger FRCS
Consultant ENT Surgeon, Plymouth General Hospital

Keith Holmes DCH CHM FRCS
Consultant Paediatric Surgeon, St George's Hospital, London

Paul Hunter MA FRCS FRCOphth
Consultant Ophthalmic Surgeon, King's College Hospital, London

Kenneth Lindsay Phd FRCS
Consultant Neurosurgeon, Southern General Hospital, Glasgow

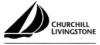

CHURCHILL
LIVINGSTONE

EDINBURGH LONDON MADRID MELBOURNE NEW YORK SAN FRANCISCO TOKYO 1996

CHURCHILL LIVINGSTONE
Medical Division of Pearson Professional Limited

Distributed in the United States of America by Churchill
Livingstone Inc., 650 Avenue of the Americas, New York,
N.Y. 10011, and by associated companies, branches and
representatives throughout the world.

First edition 1984
Second edition 1996

ISBN 0 443 048940

British Library of Cataloguing in Publication Data
A catalogue record for this book is available from the British
Library.

Library of Congress Cataloging in Publication Data
A catalog record for this book is available from the Library of
Congress.

> Medical knowledge is constantly changing. As new
> information becomes available, changes in treatment,
> procedures, equipment and the use of drugs become
> necessary. The editors, contributors and the publishers
> have, as far as it is possible, taken care to ensure that the
> information given in this text is accurate and up to date.
> However, readers are strongly advised to confirm that the
> information, especially with regard to drug usage,
> complies with current legislation and standards of
> practice.

Produced by Longman Singapore Publishers Pte Ltd
Printed in Singapore

Preface

Oral examination is a traditional and vital part of the assessment of medical students throughout their education; it allows the examiners not only to test knowledge but also to form an opinion about the candidate's ability to marshal his thoughts logically and rapidly in trying conditions. It is this immediacy that makes the clinical and viva voce parts of the final examination particularly worrying to students. There is only limited time available with teachers to practise one-to-one examination technique, so generations of students have sat at home, text books on their knees, quizzing each other. Conventional texts do not lend themselves to this process, so the authors have striven to fill the gap. We have presented surgery in an oral question and answer form, precisely as used by examiners, to help students improve their fluency and test their knowledge in a structured way.

There are some important rules to be remembered in oral examinations:

1 Listen carefully to the question — it's the only one the examiner wants answered!
2 Silence scores no points — you must start answering quickly, while remembering that you should first decide on the nub of the answer, and aim to get it across in your opening sentence.
3 Do not get bogged down in rarities and areas of controversy unless you are very sure of yourself — the examiner will know more about them than you do!

These skills only come with practice: we hope that this volume will make it easier for students to acquire them while also picking up a few extra facts. The questions and answers have been prepared by a group of surgeons who are regularly involved in teaching and yet can still remember what it is like to be on the receiving end.

London 1996

JMAN
TT
DM

Acknowledgements

We thank our wives, sons and daughters who tolerated many weekends of writing. We also thank Mrs Christine Birks for typing the manuscript.

Acknowledgements

Contents

1
Questions

'ON THE SPOT'

1   Imagine that you are faced with a 35-year-old Scottish lorry driver who has been struck down suddenly with epigastric pain which rapidly became generalized. On examination he is cold, sweaty and has abdominal rigidity and no bowel sounds.
    What would be your immediate management?

2   A child has had a tonsillectomy earlier in the day and you are called by the nurses because they suspect postoperative bleeding.
    What do you look for?

3   Imagine you are a medical houseman. A patient of yours, admitted 4 days ago with a myo-cardial infarct, develops generalized abdominal pain with guarding and loss of bowel sounds.
    What do you suspect?

4   A 75-year-old lady complains of a complete and sudden loss of her right vision 2 days previously associated with right-sided headaches for some weeks. She also admits to weight loss, anorexia and tenderness of her scalp while combing her hair.
    What steps would you take to try to ensure that she keeps her left vision?

5   You are a surgical houseman. The casualty officer refers a 2-year-old who has swallowed a penny. X-rays confirm that it is below the diaphragm.
    What are you going to do about it?

6   An obese, middle-aged man with a history of atheromatous disease presents with a 24-hour history of severe back pain. He is pale, clammy and shocked. He is too obese to confirm by palpation your suspicion of a leaking aortic aneurysm.
    What would be your further management?

7 Imagine that, as a casualty officer, you are faced with a 64-year-old man who presents in a shocked state, having developed severe left posterior chest pain while vomiting at the end of a long evening's eating and drinking. You place a calming hand on his shoulder and discover crepitus, most marked in the supraclavicular fossa.

What has happened to this man? What will the surgeons do for him?

8 An elderly patient becomes increasingly confused 3 days after major surgery.

If you were the houseman what would you do?

9 A 35-year-old alcoholic has had a large haematemesis.

What are the likely causes and how would you make the precise diagnosis?

10 What should you do during the first 24 hours following the admission of a young man who has had 3 hours of excruciating right loin pain?

11 A patient who underwent an emergency gastrectomy for perforated gastric ulcer a week ago complains of lower chest pain on inspiration and pain in the left shoulder tip. On examination he is tender under the left costal margin and has a mild pyrexia.

What may be the diagnosis and what investigations should be performed?

12 A patient becomes acutely hypotensive, breathless and unwell a week after bowel resection.

How would you sort out what is going on?

13 An old man with no past history except for rheumatoid arthritis presents with a history of vomiting a 'bucketful' of blood.

What are the principles of his management?

14 A patient with multiple injuries has a distending abdomen and frank blood is found on peritoneal lavage. However, he is unconscious due to a head injury.

Does this influence management of his abdomen?

15 A cyclist is brought into casualty after an apparently quite minor accident. By the time you see

him he is breathless and panicking.

What is your immediate management?

16 A man of 60 is taken to his family doctor having, over a period of 3 days, suffered several episodes of slurred speech and confusion from each of which he has recovered.

What is the likely cause and what must the doctor do?

17 A 4-month-old baby is brought in with a 24 hour history of intermittent screaming, pulling up of his knees, and the passage of blood and mucus per rectum.

What is the most likely diagnosis and how would you confirm it?

18 Imagine that you have admitted a patient with acute pancreatitis who fails to improve as quickly as you might normally expect. 10 days after admission, with the amylase still at 2000, you feel a mass in the epigastrium.

What do you think may be the problem? How will you confirm the diagnosis?

19 A quarryman, hurt in a rock fall, is brought to casualty. He has tried and failed to pass urine and has some blood at the urethral meatus.

What do you do next?

20 How would you manage a 60-year-old man who presents as an emergency with an episode of brisk, fresh bleeding per rectum?

21 You are the only doctor at a cardiac arrest.

What are you going to do?

22 A previously fit 60-year-old presents with weight loss, anorexia and recent, worsening dysphagia for solids.

What may be wrong? How would you investigate this patient?

23 Staff nurse bleeps you to tell you that a patient's 'bowel is in the bed'. An elderly man who had a laparotomy a week ago had a wound discharge and the registrar asked for the skin sutures to be removed.

What has happened? What will you do?

24 An elderly patient with claudication gives a few hours' history of left abdominal pain and bloody diarrhoea.
    What do you think might be wrong with him?

25 An ex-smoker is referred to outpatients with a 'groin hernia'. On examination the 'hernia' which has recently been enlarging is found to be pulsatile and to be situated close to the lower end of an axillo-femoral graft.
    What is going on? What investigations would you arrange?

26 A patient is admitted to casualty in coma following a road traffic accident.
    What are the priorities of assessment?

27 A young man, who fell on an iron spike injuring a buttock the day before, presents feeling ill and has crepitus around the wound.
    What are the likely diagnosis and management?

28 A patient complains of a painful swelling below the angle of the jaw just before meals.
    What is the likely cause?

THE ACUTE ABDOMEN

General clinical features

29 What characteristics of an abdominal pain would suggest the presence of peritoneal inflammation?

30 How does testing the urine in casualty help to make a diagnosis in a patient presenting with abdominal pain?

31 Which patients with abdominal pain experience shoulder tip pain?

32 What are the four classical symptoms of intestinal obstruction?

33 What is the difference between faecal and faeculent vomiting?

34 What is the difference between tenderness and guarding in the abdomen?

35 Which plain X-rays are usually requested on patients presenting with abdominal pain in casualty?

36 Do you know of any non-abdominal conditions which can mimic 'the acute abdomen'?

37 What acute abdominal conditions can produce back pain?

38 Why do we listen to the abdomen in patients presenting with acute abdominal pain?

Appendicitis

39 Do you know why acute appendicitis develops?

40 What are the typical symptoms and signs of appendicitis?

41 Why does the pain usually start centrally and later move to the right iliac fossa?

42 Where is McBurney's point?
   What is its significance?

43 Why is the appendix sent off for histological assessment after its surgical removal?

44 If a patient with a typical story of appendicitis is found to have a tender mass in the right iliac fossa, what may be going on?

45 What is the value of the laparoscope in managing patients with suspected appendicitis?

46 What antibiotics are routinely given before an appendicectomy and why?

Biliary disease

47 What are the typical symptoms and signs of acute cholecystitis?

48 Have you ever seen a patient with biliary colic?
   What do you remember about the clinical presentation?

49 Do you know of any investigations to help us check the diagnosis of acute cholecystitis during the acute phase?

   When is such investigation particularly important?

50 When we diagnose acute cholecystitis we give intravenous fluids and nothing by mouth.
   Why?

51 What are the indications for urgent surgery in someone with acute cholecystitis?

52 An elderly frail patient presents with jaundice and a fever — how would you manage her?

53 If you saw gas in the biliary tree on the X-rays of an old lady with unexplained small bowel obstruction, what might you suspect?

Perforated peptic ulcer

54 What does a perforated duodenal ulcer look like at operation?
   Which part of the duodenum is usually involved?

55 Why do some duodenal ulcers perforate whilst others cause bleeding?

56 Which X-ray is the most useful in the diagnosis of perforation?

57 Are any investigations required before laparotomy in a patient who clinically appears to have perforated peptic ulcer but in whom no free gas is seen on X-ray?

58 What are the usual operations for perforated duodenal or gastric ulcer?

59 Have you any idea how to manage a perforated peptic ulcer in someone medically unfit for surgery?

60 Do you know of any drugs that predispose to perforated peptic ulcer?

Complications of diverticular disease

61 What is the difference between diverticulosis and diverticulitis?

62 What do we mean by 'left-sided appendicitis'?

63 How is acute diverticulitis diagnosed and managed?

64 What are the clinical features of pericolic abscess? How is it managed?

65 An old man with a long history of diverticular disease has suffered repeated attacks of rigors and dysuria over the past few months.
   What may be going on?

66 What is the Hartmann procedure and when is it used for diverticular disease?

67 What is the prognosis in patients suffering from perforated diverticular disease?

Acute pancreatitis

68 What are the causes of acute pancreatitis?

69 What are the typical clinical features of this condition?

70 How do you confirm the diagnosis?

71 How would you manage a patient with this condition?

72 How do you assess the severity of an attack of acute pancreatitis?

Vascular conditions

73 What part of the bowel is usually affected by embolic mesenteric infarction? Is this condition treatable?

74 What will help you to make a diagnosis of acute mesenteric infarction?

75 What are the typical features of a leaking aortic aneurysm?
   What may it mimic?

76 Does ischaemic colitis usually require operation?

Gynaecological conditions

77 What gynaecological emergencies can mimic appendicitis?

78 Do you know how a ruptured ectopic pregnancy presents?

79 How would you distinguish between appendicitis and acute salpingitis?

Intestinal obstruction

80 What are the commonest causes of small bowel obstruction in adults?

81 Why do patients with distal small bowel obstruction become dehydrated, even before they have started vomiting?

82 What do we mean by reversed peristalsis?

83 What is closed-loop obstruction?

84 What is subacute obstruction?

85 How do we go about deciding how much and what type of intravenous fluid replacement to give to a patient with intestinal obstruction?

86 What are the constituents of 'normal' saline?

87 What is Hartmann's solution?

88 How do we differentiate small bowel from large bowel in the abdominal X-rays of someone with intestinal obstruction?
   Why do we bother?

89 What blood tests would you order in someone with intestinal obstruction?

90 Following a total hip replacement a patient develops vomiting and abdominal distension.
What would you suspect and how would you confirm the diagnosis?

91 Is visible peristalsis always pathological?

92 What sort of acid-base abnormality develops in intestinal obstruction?

93 What X-ray signs would indicate the presence of dead bowel in someone with intestinal obstruction?

94 What radiological investigations might you order in a child with a suspected ileocolic intussusception?

95 What are the commonest abdominal operations leading to adhesions and hence adhesive small bowel obstruction?

96 How do we decide if and when to operate on someone with small bowel obstruction due to adhesions?

97 Why are colostomies and ileostomies sometimes fashioned in patients with obstruction?

98 Are there any types of small bowel obstruction peculiar to patients who have previously undergone a gastrectomy?

99 What are the major worries for an anaesthetist preparing a patient with acute intestinal obstruction for operation?

100 What symptoms and signs suggest that someone with small bowel obstruction has developed strangulation of a bowel segment?

101 How do the symptoms of small and large bowel obstruction differ?

102 What is the commonest cause of large bowel obstruction?

103 What is spurious diarrhoea?

104 Are there any dangers in 'sitting on' a case of large bowel obstruction?

105 What is sigmoid volvulus?

106 How do we treat someone with intestinal obstruction due to sigmoid carcinoma?

107 In what conditions may dilated bowel be seen on a plain abdominal X-ray without there being any mechanical obstruction to the passage of bowel contents?

108 What is a 'string' carcinoma?

Abdominal trauma

109 An unconscious man who is hypotensive after a head injury is noted to have an abdominal bruise. How should he be managed?

110 What symptoms and signs suggest the diagnosis of ruptured spleen?

111 Why may surgeons try to preserve the spleen if it is injured?

112 Why does a chest wall injury in a road traffic accident patient make evaluation of abdominal signs more difficult?

113 Up to what level on the chest wall should penetrating injuries be regarded as having possibly entered the abdominal cavity?

114 What intra-abdominal organs are specially liable to injury in a patient wearing a seat-belt during a head-on collision?

115 What are the relative dangers of intra-abdominal visceral damage due to injuries produced by a knife, hand-gun and high-velocity rifle?

116 Following a stabbing, the victim is found at laparotomy to have a knife wound in the anterior wall of the stomach. The surgeon simply repairs this and closes the abdomen.
    He is likely to be re-operating soon — why?

117 What is a subcapsular haematoma of the spleen? What is its significance?

118 How can a crush injury to the abdomen result in severe mechanical respiratory embarrassment?

119 What is the most efficient investigation to check for intraperitoneal haemorrhage? What are the contraindications?

120 What are the radiological signs of a ruptured spleen?

121 What is the usefulness of inserting a probe into an abdominal stab wound to assess the depth of penetration?

122 What X-ray signs suggest a diaphragmatic rupture?

123 In which types of abdominal trauma is laparotomy mandatory?

124 How would you manage a patient admitted with abdominal trauma in whom laparotomy is not immediately indicated?

125 How would you manage a patient with a knife wound to the abdomen?

126 What antibiotics would you prescribe as part of the treatment of a patient with a stab wound involving the large bowel?

127 A patient who has received a stab wound to the abdomen is found at laparotomy to have a laceration of the right lobe of the liver. What surgical manoeuvres are likely to be considered?

GENERAL SURGICAL CARE

Water, electrolytes and nutrition

128 What are the body's normal daily gains and losses of water?

129 How would you assess the water requirements of a patient in the first 24 hours after a routine abdominal operation?

130 You may have to repeat the exercise on a more complicated, critically ill patient.
   What other factors should be taken into account?

131 What is the normal 24 hour turnover of sodium?

132 How would you interpret a serum sodium of 124 mmol/litre?

133 What is the significance of a high serum sodium?

134 How much potassium is contained in the urine?

135 How might a low serum potassium occur?
   What are the possible consequences?

136 A patient's potassium rises to 6.8 mmol/litre after surgery.
   What are you going to do about it?

137 In a patient with intestinal obstruction and a Ryle's tube down, what approximate electrolyte composition would you expect in the aspirate?
   How would you take account of this in your fluid replacement?

138 How would you judge the appropriate intravenous replacement for the loss from a gastro-intestinal fistula?

139 What hazards may be encountered in the treatment of hypokalaemia?

140 In what chemical forms is calcium found in serum?

141 Suggest some causes for and consequences of hypercalcaemia.

142 Under what circumstances may magnesium deficiency occur?

143 What surgical problems may be encountered in a patient who has had difficulty taking an adequate diet in the pre-operative period?

144　If it proves necessary to maintain a patient by the intravenous route alone, what basic constituents should this diet contain?

145　What risks are entailed in this therapy?

Management of the circulation

146　What do you understand by the term 'shock'?

147　Define 'hypovolaemia' and explain how you would reach this diagnosis.

148　What solutions are available for expanding the circulation and what are their relative merits?

149　What information can you gain by measuring the central venous pressure?

150　How would you set about measuring the central venous pressure?

151　How would you define oliguria?

152　What immediate steps would you take to remedy oliguria?

153　What factors cause or contribute to the development of acute renal failure?

154　How would you manage this condition?

155　Soon after a major operation your patient is noted to have a diastolic blood pressure of 110 mmHg. How do you assess and manage this?

156　Summarize the potential hazards of blood transfusion.

157　The patient is bleeding excessively during surgery and you suspect a coagulopathy. How do you confirm and manage the problem?

Postoperative complications

158　List some possible causes of a pyrexia noted between 3 and 10 days after surgery.

159 How would you investigate a low grade pyrexia during the week after surgery for which the cause is not obvious?

160 What are the implications of a swinging pyrexia during the second week after an abdominal operation?

161 What factors contribute to the occurrence of wound infections?

162 What organisms would you specifically enquire about in infection complicating a large bowel resection?

163 If you have located an abscess and know the organism, how would you treat it?

164 What pulmonary complications might be anticipated after major surgery?

165 What precautions can be taken to reduce the potential chest problems in a bronchitic undergoing abdominal surgery?

166 What is intrapulmonary shunting?
How would you recognize and deal with it?

167 In the second postoperative week a patient coughs up some blood.
What steps would you take?

168 What is Virchow's triad?
How does it apply to the postoperative patient?

169 Why would you suspect and how would you confirm the diagnosis of a deep vein thrombosis?

170 When and how would you anticoagulate a patient following a deep vein thrombosis?

171 What are the typical clinical features of pulmonary embolism?
How would you confirm the diagnosis?

172 What treatment is available?

173 How do we try to prevent thrombo-embolism?

174 If a myocardial infarction occurs under anaesthetic, the typical clinical features are not seen. How would you know it had happened?

175 The night of the operation a tachycardia is noted. How would you decide what to do about it?

176 Define primary, secondary and reactionary haemorrhage.

177 How would you deal with sudden profuse bleeding from an abdominal drain?

'LUMPS AND BUMPS'

178 In your examination of a lump what physical features would you note?

179 How would you elicit fluctuance?

180 What would you infer if the lump were tethered?

181 How would tensing the muscles in the region of a lump help decide its anatomical position?

182 What features of a lump permit transillumination?

183 What general features would suggest bacterial infection as the cause of a lump?

184 How is an abscess diagnosed and managed?

185 What is cellulitis and what organism is likely to be responsible?

186 What is the difference between a boil and a carbuncle?

187 What is the likely nature of a soft, lobulated, subcutaneous lump?

188 What is Dercum's disease?

189 What are the typical clinical features of a sebaceous cyst?

190 What causes warts to come and go?

191 What is keloid?

192 Outline the essentials of the TNM classification of malignant tumours.

193 What changes in a mole make malignancy a possibility?

194 How would you confirm the diagnosis in a clinically suspected malignant melanoma?

195 What factors may predispose to squamous cell carcinoma?

196 Describe the clinical features of a rodent ulcer.

197 Give the differential diagnosis in a patient who is found to have enlarged axillary lymph nodes.

198 A patient reports that he develops a swelling in his neck immediately after eating.
    What might it be?

199 A group of enlarged nodes is found on one side of the neck.
    What are the possible diagnoses?

200 A recently noticed tender lump in the groin might be due to what?

201 What do you think was particularly important about the original description of Burkitt's tumour?

202 What are the causes of a tender scrotal swelling?

HERNIA

203 What are the surface landmarks of the superficial inguinal ring?

204 What are the boundaries of the deep inguinal ring?

205 What structures constitute the spermatic cord?

206 What are the boundaries of the femoral canal?

207 Define the term 'hernia'.

208 What is the importance of the neck of a hernial sac?

209 What types of hernia occur in the groin?

210 Explain the exact meaning of the words 'direct' and 'indirect' in this context.

211 Can you give the relative frequency of the various types of groin hernia?

212 What would you include in the differential diagnosis of inguinoscrotal swellings in children?

213 Which inguinal herniae can be considered more likely to be congenital and which to be acquired?

214 How often are groin herniae bilateral?

215 On the grounds of probability alone, what type of groin hernia are you most likely to find in a woman?

216 Besides the groin, where else may an external hernia occur?

217 What is meant by the word 'exomphalos'?

218 What is the usual outcome of an umbilical hernia noted soon after birth?

219 What is the aetiology of incisional hernia and how may it be avoided?

220 What exactly is meant by the term 'herniotomy'?

221 What are the principles involved in the repair of adult inguinal herniae?

222 Explain what is meant by a sliding hernia. What is its other name?

223 What is the difference between umbilical and paraumbilical herniae?

224 Is surgery always successful in the repair of inguinal hernia?

225 How may a femoral hernia be differentiated from an enlarged lymph node at the same site?

226 Explain the meaning of strangulation, obstruction, incarceration and irreducibility as applied to a hernia.

227 Of the groin herniae, which are the more liable to strangulate?

228 What complications may occur with a femoral hernia?

229 Describe some eponymous herniae.

230 In what circumstances can strangulation occur without obstruction?

231 How do you decide which hernia patients can be treated as day cases?

232 How long should a patient take off work after a hernia repair? When can they start driving?

ALIMENTARY TRACT (EXCLUDING LARGE BOWEL)

The mouth and salivary glands

233 An old lady who has recently undergone major surgery complains of a sore mouth. On examination she has many white patches on the lining of the buccal cavity.
   What are the diagnosis and management?

234 What are the typical symptoms and signs of cancer of the tongue?

235 What is meant by a tongue tie?

236 What is the cause of a mucus retention cyst and how should it be treated?

237 An old man develops a painful, brawny red swelling on one side of his face in front of the ear several days after a major abdominal operation.
   What is the most likely diagnosis? Why does this condition develop?

238 What nerves are liable to damage during surgery on the salivary glands?

239 Where do the parotid and submandibular salivary ducts open into the mouth?

240 Why is mumps parotitis so painful?

241 What are the various names of the commonest tumour of the parotid gland?
     How is it treated?

242 What are the chances of recurrence after removal of a pleomorphic adenoma of the parotid?

243 What medical conditions can cause salivary gland enlargement?

244 What is thought to be the cause of salivary duct stones?

245 How do we manage a patient with a submandibular duct stone?

The oesophagus

246 What anatomical factors normally prevent reflux at the lower end of the oesophagus?

247 What are the structures of the oesophageal wall?

248 Define dysphagia.
     List some causes.

249 A barium swallow in a patient with dysphagia shows an 'apple core' lesion.
     What other tests are required to decide on appropriate treatment?

250 How can potassium therapy cause an oesophageal stricture?

251 Briefly, what do you know of the pathology of oesophageal cancer?

252 How can a tumour of the oesophagus be treated without opening the chest?

253 What is the prognosis in patients with carcinoma of the oesophagus?

254 What is heartburn?
How would you advise a patient with this symptom?

255 What sorts of hiatal herniae do you know?
How may their presentation differ?

256 What complications can develop in patients with sliding hiatal hernia?

257 Can you list the indications and types of surgical treatment available for reflux oesophagitis?

258 What do you know about achalasia?

259 Where exactly do benign oesophageal strictures usually occur?
How are they managed?

260 What forms of treatment are available for bleeding oesophageal varices?

The stomach

261 What structures related to the stomach may become involved by direct spread of a gastric cancer?

262 What is the blood supply of the stomach?

263 What are the functions of the stomach?

264 What parts of the stomach produce gastrin, acid and pepsin?

265 What stimuli induce gastric acid secretion?

266 How can we reduce gastric acid secretion?

267 What are the different ways in which gastric cancer can present?

268 Do you know any factors which predispose to gastric cancer?

269 What are 'hour glass' and 'leather bottle' stomachs?

270 Briefly, what operations are available for gastric cancer?

271 Can we offer patients with gastric cancer a good chance of cure?

272 Why do patients with gastric ulcer tend to lose weight?

273 In a patient with a gastric ulcer what is the significance of back pain?

274 Why should gastroscopy be mandatory in the investigation of a gastric ulcer patient?

275 How should we manage a patient with an apparently benign, uncomplicated gastric ulcer?

276 What are the complications of gastric ulcer?

277 What radiological features suggest a gastric ulcer might be malignant?

278 What is erosive gastritis?
    What are its causes?

279 How do we manage a patient who is shown endoscopically to be bleeding from erosive gastritis?

280 What are the important causes of upper gastro-intestinal bleeding?

281 Why do most clinicians prefer to endoscope patients with upper gastro-intestinal bleeding soon after admission?
    Does this investigation affect mortality?

282 What sorts of treatment are available for bleeding peptic ulcers (gastric and duodenal)?

283 Why do patients become anaemic after gastrectomy?

The duodenum

284 What structures may be involved when a duodenal ulcer penetrates through the wall?

285 What is the significance of a duodenal diverticulum?

286 What hormones does the duodenal mucosa secrete? What stimulates their production and what are their actions?

287 How is the duodenal mucosa normally protected from acid/peptic digestion?

288 What may be the relationship between *Helicobacter pylorii* and duodenal ulcers?
   How do we demonstrate its presence in a patient with a duodenal ulcer?

289 How does a duodenal ulcer usually present?

290 Why do some patients with duodenal ulcers bleed and others perforate?

291 What is the first line treatment in the patient with a simple duodenal ulcer?

292 When and how do you treat *Helicobacter pylorii*?

293 What are the indications for surgery in duodenal ulcer?

294 What operations are available for duodenal ulcer?

295 What is meant by a pyloroplasty?
   When is it used and what are the alternatives?

296 What are the long-term complications of duodenal ulcer surgery?

The pancreas

297 What is the nerve supply of the pancreas?
   When is this clinically important?

298 How is pancreatic exocrine function controlled?

299 What tumours may occur in the pancreas?

300 How does the presentation of cancer of the head of the pancreas differ from that of cancer of the body or tail?

301 Can we prove a diagnosis of pancreatic cancer without laparotomy?

302 When is a Whipple's operation performed?
    Why has it fallen into disfavour?

303 What is chronic pancreatitis?

304 What forms of treatment are available for chronic
    pancreatitis?

305 What is a pancreatic pseudocyst?
    How is it managed?

The liver

306 Describe the anatomical divisions of the liver.
    What is their clinical relevance?

307 What structures are in danger of accidental dam-
    age during an attempted liver biopsy?

308 How can we diagnose liver secondaries?

309 Are liver secondaries treatable?
    If so, how?

310 What are the conditions known to predispose to
    primary hepatocellular carcinoma?

311 What liver condition is particularly related to con-
    tact with sheep?

312 Who gets liver abscesses in this country?

313 How can we treat a unilocular liver abscess?

314 How may the surgeon become involved in the
    management of cirrhosis?

315 What are the indications for liver transplantation?
    What does the operation involve?

The biliary tree

316 What anatomical structures are at risk of acciden-
    tal damage during cholecystectomy?
    How do such injuries occur?

317 What is the anatomy of the lower end of the common bile duct?

318 What are the functions of bile? *Exo eacretory*

319 What incidental lesions may be found on ultrasound of the biliary tree?

320 What abnormalities of bile lead to stone formation?

321 Can you describe the typical 'gall-stone patient' and her symptoms?

322 What are the complications of gall-stones?

323 What investigations help confirm the clinical suspicion of gall-bladder disease?
How are they performed?

324 What is Courvoisier's Law and what is its use?

325 What are the surgical approaches and their relative indications for removal of the gall-bladder?

326 What is operative cholangiography?

327 Can stones be 'removed' from the gall-bladder other than by surgery?

328 What do we mean by obstructive jaundice?
What are the causes?

329 Why do patients with obstructive jaundice often complain of itching?
How can it be treated?

330 How do we confirm obstructive jaundice biochemically?

331 What are the options for treatment of obstructive jaundice due to gall-stones?

332 What is the hepatorenal syndrome and how do we try to prevent it?

333 What is a T-tube?
How do we manage it postoperatively?

334 What is a mucocele of the gall-bladder?

335 What are the causes of bile duct strictures?

336 What do you know about gall-bladder cancer?

The spleen

337 What organs may be damaged during splenectomy?

338 How may an enlarged spleen be differentiated from an enlarged kidney?

339 What are the commonest causes of splenomegaly in Europe?

340 What are the usual indications for splenectomy?

341 What are the early and late complications of splenectomy?

342 What is the difference between splenomegaly and hypersplenism?

The small bowel

343 What major artery supplies the small bowel?
   What is the course of the trunk of this vessel?

344 What are the physiological consequences of resection of the distal 60 cm of ileum?

345 How does Crohn's disease affecting the small bowel usually present?

346 What are the extra-abdominal GI manifestations of Crohn's disease?

347 What are the radiological characteristics of Crohn's disease?

348 What are the indications for surgery in Crohn's disease?

349 What is intussusception?
   What causes it?

350 How can a Meckel's diverticulum make its owner acutely ill?

351 How may a patient with radiation damage to the small bowel present?

352 Why is an ileostomy made the way it is?
     What is it like to have one?

The peritoneal cavity

353 How do you diagnose ascites and what are the major causes?

354 How can we treat malignant ascites?

355 What are the causes of pelvic abscess?
     How is it diagnosed and treated?

356 What do you know about pseudomyxoma peritonei?

The large bowel

357 Briefly, what is the blood supply of the large bowel?

358 What anatomical features determine that diverticular disease affects the colon, but not the rectum?

359 What structures may be damaged during mobilization of the bowel for a right hemicolectomy?

360 What are the physiological functions of the large bowel?

361 What do you know about the relationship between diet and colorectal cancer?

362 Do you know of any inherited abnormalities which predispose to colorectal cancer?

363 What is screening, and when should it be used?
     How might we screen the population for colorectal cancer?

364 Which parts of the large bowel are most frequently affected by carcinoma?

365 How do the classical symptoms of right- and left-sided colonic cancer differ?

366 How would you investigate an adult complaining of the passage of blood and mucus per rectum?

367 What are the basic principles for deciding the extent of a radical operation for large bowel cancer?

368 What is the Dukes' staging system for large bowel cancer?
  What is its prognostic significance?

369 What large bowel conditions are premalignant?

370 What arterial or cardiac diseases may affect the large bowel?

371 What do you know about the pathophysiology of diverticular disease of the colon?
  How common is colonic diverticular disease?

372 How does colonic diverticular disease most commonly present?

373 What advice would you give to a patient who has been shown to have uncomplicated colonic diverticular disease?

374 What are the complications of colonic diverticular disease?
  Why do they develop?

375 A man of 60 presents with a history of bleeding and mucus per rectum. Sigmoidoscopy is normal, a barium enema shows diverticular disease.
  Where do we go from here?

376 What types of rectal prolapse do you know?
  What groups develop this condition?

377 How can we treat complete rectal prolapse in an otherwise fit 70-year-old?

378 What are the complications of ulcerative colitis?

379 What are the indications for surgery in ulcerative colitis?
  What are the usual surgical procedures?

380 How often does Crohn's disease affect the large bowel?
   What are its clinical manifestations?

381 What drugs are available for the treatment of ulcerative colitis?
   How effective are they in patients with Crohn's disease?

382 Is surgery often needed for patients with brisk bleeding per rectum?
   What investigations should be carried out pre-operatively?

383 A 25-year-old woman presents with several years' history of griping abdominal pain, bloating of the abdomen and an irregular bowel habit.
   What is the most likely diagnosis, and how can we be sure that this is the cause of her symptoms?

384 What symptoms may be caused by colorectal polyps?
   How can we remove these lesions?

The anus and anal canal

385 Which part of the anal sphincter is vital for faecal continence?

386 What lines the anal canal?

387 How do you perform a digital examination of the anus and rectum?

388 What are the typical symptoms of piles?

389 What investigations should be carried out before we assume a patient's piles are the cause of his complaint of rectal bleeding?

390 How do we classify piles?
   How does the treatment of piles vary with their extent?

391 What would you do, as a surgical houseman, if a patient began to bleed from the operation site several hours after haemorrhoidectomy?

392 What is an anal fissure?
What symptoms and signs does it produce?

393 What is a fistula-in-ano?
How do we diagnose it?

394 How do we treat a fistula-in-ano?
What are the dangers of operation?

395 Abscesses around the anal region are sometimes associated with more generalized diseases.
Can you name some?

396 What are the more important causes of faecal incontinence in women?

397 What measures are available to help a patient suffering from faecal incontinence due to a sphincter deficiency?

398 What do you know of the types and mode of spread of cancer of the anus and anal canal?

399 Do you know any sexually transmitted diseases (STDs) which may affect the anus?

400 What is a perianal haematoma and how does it present?

THE BREAST

401 What is the lymphatic drainage of the breast?

402 A woman complains of a discharge from the nipple.
What would reassure you that there was no serious cause for it?

403 Why might a patient presenting with a breast lump also complain of increasing breathlessness?

404 What features in a breast lump might suggest that it is malignant?

405 What is the difference between skin tethering and skin fixity of a breast lump?

406 An old lady presents complaining that one breast has become much smaller than the other and the nipple replaced by a scab.
What is the probable diagnosis?

407 What is the importance of nipple inversion?

408 What is Paget's disease of the nipple?

409 What is peau d'orange?

410 Why may the arm become swollen in breast cancer patients?

411 What are the roles of mammography?

412 What are the radiological signs of a breast carcinoma on a mammogram?

413 In which population groups is breast cancer screening appropriate?

414 What sorts of radiological investigation help us assess a patient who may have breast cancer?

415 What is the prognostic importance of axillary lymph node involvement in a case of breast cancer?

416 What are the commonest sites of distant spread in breast cancer?

417 Do you know anything about the different theories on how breast cancer metastasizes?
How does this problem affect our approach to treatment?

418 How is a guide wire excision of an area of microcalcification performed?

419 Which patients with breast cancer need a mastectomy?

420 Define 'simple' and 'radical' mastectomies.

421 What part does radiotherapy play in the treatment of early breast cancer?

422 How do we deal with the cosmetic deformity produced by mastectomy?

423 What patterns of advanced breast cancer do you know of?

424 Does surgery have any part to play in the treatment of advanced breast cancer?

425 How do bone metastases present in breast cancer?
How do we treat them?

426 What sorts of endocrine therapy do we use in advanced breast cancer?
How do we choose the therapy for a particular patient?

427 A woman who has had a breast carcinoma is concerned that she might develop one in the other breast.
What would you tell her?

428 What is a 'breast mouse'?

429 What physical signs would suggest to you that a breast lump is a simple cyst?

430 Generalized 'lumpiness' in the breasts, with or without pain, is sometimes encountered.
What is the usual cause?

431 How may an intraduct papilloma present?

432 How is fine needle aspiration cytology performed?
What is its value?

433 As a rule what is the safe course in the treatment of a breast cyst that hasn't disappeared completely on aspiration?

434 What can be done for a woman with intermittently painful breasts?

435 What is the histology of a fibro-adenoma?

436 Do you know of any benign breast disease that clinically may mimic cancer?

437 Which groups are liable to develop breast abscess?

438 What clinical features suggest breast abscess?

439 A mother who is breast feeding suddenly develops a painful lump in her breast.
How would you manage her?

440 What is the surgical treatment of a breast abscess?
What organisms may be cultured from the pus?

441 What is cyclical mastalgia and how can it be treated?

442 What is gynaecomastia?
Does it require treatment?

443 Why might a plastic surgeon operate on the breast?

THE ENDOCRINE SYSTEM

444 How does the thyroid gland develop?
What abnormalities of development can occur?

445 How does the thyroid gland produce T3 and T4?

446 What tests can be performed to assess thyroid function?

447 What may be the significance of a 'cold nodule' on a radio-isotope thyroid scan?

448 What are the causes of a non-toxic goitre?

449 What is the value of fine needle aspiration cytology in the management of thyroid swellings?

450 List the possible causes of thyrotoxicosis.

451 Describe the symptoms and signs of Graves' disease.

452 How do antithyroid drugs work?
Which are used most frequently?

453 In which patients is radioactive iodine used for treatment of thyrotoxicosis, and how effective is it?

454 What are the indications for surgery in thyrotoxicosis?

455 How is a thyrotoxic patient prepared for surgery?

456 What is the significance of an apparently solitary thyroid nodule?

457 Why is surgery performed in patients with nodular goitre?

458 What are the specific complications of thyroid-ectomy?

459 List the main types of thyroid carcinoma.

460 Why do we check the vocal cords before doing a thyroidectomy?

461 Compare the clinical and histological features of papillary and follicular carcinoma of the thyroid.

462 How does the treatment of thyroid cancer depend on the histological type?

463 What are the various forms of thyroiditis?

464 Outline the clinical features of Hashimoto's thyroiditis.
How is the diagnosis confirmed and the condition treated?

465 How do the parathyroid glands develop?
How are they identified at operation?

466 What are the causes of hyperparathyroidism?

467 In what ways may hyperparathyroidism present?

468 How is the diagnosis of primary hyperpara-thyroidism confirmed?

469 Following parathyroidectomy, hypocalcaemia may occur.
How is this recognized and treated?

470 What are the causes of Cushing's syndrome?

471 What are the typical features of Cushing's syn-drome?

472 How is Cushing's syndrome due to a pituitary tu-mour treated?

473 What is the underlying abnormality in Conn's syndrome?
    How does it affect the patient?

474 Which patients might benefit from adrenalectomy?

THE ARTERIES, VEINS AND LYMPHATICS

475 There are two main symptoms of peripheral vascular disease in the legs.
    What are they and what is their significance?

476 What is the natural history of intermittent claudication?

477 Why is rest pain worse at night?

478 A patient complains of buttock pain on walking and impotence, what is the likely diagnosis?

479 Atherosclerosis affects particular sites in the peripheral vascular system.
    What are they?

480 What conditions can mimic intermittent claudication?

481 What are the major items in the examination of a patient with peripheral vascular disease in the legs?

482 What is the significance of a femoral bruit?

483 What general advice can be given to patients with peripheral vascular disease?

484 How can peripheral vascular disease be assessed with non-invasive tests?

485 What is meant by the 'ankle/brachial pressure index' and how is it interpreted?

486 In which patients with peripheral vascular disease should angiography be performed?

487 How can angiography be performed?

488 Describe the typical pathological features of atherosclerosis.

489 Why does atheroma develop?

490 What non-operative treatment may be tried in patients with peripheral vascular disease?

491 How can a lumbar sympathectomy be performed?
What does it achieve?

492 Why may diabetics get problems with their feet?

493 List the causes of acute ischaemia of the leg.

494 What are the different types of material available for arterial grafts?

495 What is meant by angioplasty?
How is this performed?

496 What are extra-anatomic grafts?

497 Where does atheroma usually affect the superficial femoral artery?

498 What is a trouser graft and when is it used?

499 How much does an artery need to be narrowed before there is a significant reduction in flow?

500 How may an occluded superficial femoral artery be bypassed?

501 What factors are involved with the long-term patency of grafts?

502 What are the indications for amputation in peripheral vascular disease?
What principles determine the level of amputation?

503 What is an aneurysm?
List the various types.

504 What is a false aneurysm?
How does it develop?

505 What is an aortic dissection?

506 How may an aortic dissection present?

507 When is surgery indicated for aortic dissection?

508 How can an abdominal aortic aneurysm present?

509 Outline how a patient with an unruptured abdominal aortic aneurysm should be managed.

510 Should patients with asymptomatic aortic aneurysms have elective surgery?

511 Are all abdominal aortic aneurysms resectable?
    Are there any other methods of treatment?

512 Where can peripheral aneurysms occur?
    Who first described their surgical treatment?

513 Define an embolus and list the various types.

514 Where do peripheral arterial emboli usually lodge and what effects do they produce?

515 What does a lower limb embolectomy involve?

516 What are streptokinase and TPA?
    How can they be used in the treatment of acute arterial occlusion?

517 What is Buerger's disease?

518 Why may a surgeon be asked to see a case of suspected temporal arteritis urgently?

519 What is Raynaud's phenomenon?

520 In which conditions may Raynaud's phenomenon occur?

521 What is Raynaud's disease?

522 How may atheroma of the carotid artery present?

523 What is the natural history of an asymptomatic carotid bruit?

524 Outline the ways in which carotid artery atheroma is assessed.

525 Have anti-platelet drugs been shown to be of value in carotid atheroma?

526 What are the indications for operating on patients suffering from transient ischaemic attacks?

527 What is the subclavian steal syndrome?

528 How may acute mesenteric ischaemia present?

529 Ischaemic colitis produces typical radiographic appearances.
   What are they?

530 What clinical features are associated with chronic mesenteric ischaemia?

531 What is a carotid body tumour?

532 Do we know why varicose veins develop?

533 How would you examine a patient with varicose veins?

534 Compare the non-operative and operative treatment of varicose veins.

535 What is the difference between stripping and avulsion of varicose veins?

536 What are the causes of venous ulcers?
   How may they be treated?

537 What is thrombophlebitis?
   How should it be managed?

538 What is varicose eczema?

BURNS

539 In the assessment of the area of a burn what is the 'rule of nines'?

540 Why is it important to assess the area and depth of burns?

541 What do the initials ATLS stand for and what is their connection with the management of burns?

542 Why do burn patients become dehydrated, and how do we minimize this problem?

543 How may renal failure develop in burn patients?

544 How widespread must a burn be before IV fluid is required?

545 What are the immediate steps in the management of the badly burned patient?

546 How do we assess the fluid replacement required in a burn patient?

547 When is blood transfusion required after a burn?

548 How do we assess the depth of a burn?

549 What parameters are monitored during the treatment of a badly burned patient?

550 When are skin grafts required in burn patients?
Why are they used?

551 How do we prepare and apply skin grafts in the burn patient?

552 What are the major causes of death in burn patients?

553 How do we routinely try to prevent infection of burns?
What are the important organisms involved?

554 What is the recommended treatment for someone who runs from a blazing building with their clothes on fire?

555 What injuries does lightning cause?

556 Which patients should be referred to specialized burns units?

557 Which burn patients are likely to suffer lung damage?
How should this be managed?

558   Should an asymptomatic inguinal hernia be oper-
      ated on in the first year of life?

559   How is an obstructed or incarcerated hernia
      treated in a baby?

560   What is an umbilical hernia?
          How is it managed?

561   Name the two congenital abdominal wall defects
      and list the important differences between them.

562   What features suggest oesophageal atresia in a
      neonate and how does this and a commonly asso-
      ciated abnormality threaten life?

563   How may gastro-oesophageal reflux present in
      childhood?

564   How is gastro-oesophageal reflux assessed and
      treated?

565   List the causes of neonatal intestinal obstruction.

566   What are the symptoms and signs of neonatal
      intestinal obstruction?

567   What are the indications for circumcision in a
      child?

568   Why is inspection of the anus an important part
      of neonatal examination?

569   What are the characteristic features of infantile
      pyloric stenosis?

570   What is the name of the operation for this condi-
      tion and what does it involve?

571   What are the characteristic features of intus-
      susception?

572   How would you confirm the presence of and treat
      intussusception in a child?

573 What are the commoner causes of rectal bleeding in childhood?

574 How do we manage a child who has swallowed a foreign body?

575 What are hypospadias and epispadias?

576 What are the features of an infantile hydrocele and how is it treated?

577 By what age should testicular descent have occurred?

578 What is the most common explanation for an empty scrotum?

579 List the commoner solid tumours of childhood.

580 What are the principles of treating childhood tumours?

THE GENITO-URINARY SYSTEM

General points

581 What different types of pain are associated with urinary tract disease?

582 List the causes of haematuria.

583 How does the timing of haematuria in relation to micturition aid differential diagnosis?

584 If haematuria follows insignificant renal trauma what might it suggest?

585 Why is a neurological examination an essential part of a urological assessment?

586 By what criteria can a urinary infection be diagnosed in a urine sample?

587 What is sterile pyuria?
      What are its main causes?

588 How is an intravenous urogram performed and what information can it provide?

589 What are the causes of calculi in the urinary tract?

590 List the types and appearances of urinary tract calculi.

591 Classify renal failure.

592 What features would suggest that renal failure might be due to obstruction in the urinary tract?

593 What is pneumaturia?
Outline its causes.

The kidney and ureter

594 Compare the physical signs of renal and splenic enlargement.

595 What simple tests of renal function are commonly used?

596 List the common congenital renal anomalies.

597 What investigation is most useful in determining obstruction to a kidney?
What other information can this investigation provide?

598 Why is an intravenous urogram of importance in the management of renal trauma?

599 What are the indications for surgical intervention in the management of renal trauma?

600 List the typical clinical and pathological features of acute pyelonephritis.

601 What is a JJ stent and in what circumstances might it be used?

602 What are the indications for open surgery for stones in the kidney or upper ureter?

603 What are pyonephrosis and perinephric abscess?

604 What types of lithotripter are now available?

605 What is meant by percutaneous nephrolithotomy and how is it performed?

606 Which urinary calculi are radiolucent?
What percentage of all urinary calculi do these represent?

607 Classify renal tumours.

608 How may patients with renal cell carcinoma present?

609 How are renal tumours in adults treated?

610 What is the importance of tissue typing in renal transplantation?

611 Compare the results of cadaveric and live-related donor renal transplantation.

612 How is immunosuppression used following renal transplantation?

613 What are the common complications of renal transplantation?

614 What do we mean by a duplex collecting system?

615 List the causes of bilateral hydronephrosis.

616 How is suspected pelvi-ureteric junction obstruction diagnosed and treated?

617 How would you manage a patient with suspected ureteric colic?

618 How could a 1cm stone in the upper ureter be treated?

619 What are the indications for surgery in ureteric calculi?

620 Define retroperitoneal fibrosis and list the causes.

621 List the commoner causes of ureteric injury.

622 What is vesico-ureteric reflux?
How is it diagnosed?

623 How should a patient with reflux be managed?

The bladder, prostate and urethra

624   What symptoms may a patient with bladder out-flow obstruction have?

625   What are the causes of cystitis?

626   What is interstitial cystitis and how may it be treated?

627   What are the effects of prostatic enlargement on the bladder?

628   Which agents can induce malignant change in the urothelium?

629   List the common presentations of carcinoma of the bladder.

630   What types of bladder carcinoma occur?

631   How is carcinoma of the bladder diagnosed and staged?

632   How is bladder cancer treated?

633   What is an ileal conduit?

634   Why may bladder diverticula develop?
      What are their complications?

635   Define urinary incontinence and enuresis.

636   How may urodynamic studies help in the investigation of incontinence?

637   What are the principles in the management of incontinence?

638   Compare acute and chronic urinary retention.

639   List the causes of acute urinary retention.

640   How should acute postoperative retention be managed?

641   What may happen if a chronically distended bladder is decompressed too rapidly?

642 Outline the risks of prolonged catheterization. How may these be minimized?

643 How should patients with acute urinary retention be prepared for surgery?

644 What information about the prostate may be revealed by a rectal examination?

645 What methods — other than prostatectomy — are available for the treatment of bladder outflow obstruction due to prostatic hypertrophy?

646 What is prostatitis and what are the different types?

647 What is the significance of residual urine?

648 List the indications for prostatectomy.

649 How may prostatectomy be performed? What does it aim to achieve?

650 What are the complications of prostatectomy?

651 How does carcinoma of the prostate present?

652 How do we diagnose and stage prostatic carcinoma?

653 How may carcinoma of the prostate be treated?

654 What methods are available for hormonal manipulations in the treatment of carcinoma of the prostate?

655 What are the causes of urethral stricture?

656 What are the different parts of the urethra and which are most vulnerable to injury?

657 How does membranous urethral injury occur? What are its effects?

658 How may a patient with a suspected urethral stricture be investigated and treated?

The male genitalia

659 What may cause an enlargement of the testes?

660 What do you know about the aetiology of epididymo-orchitis?

661 How do you tell the difference between acute epididymo-orchitis and testicular torsion?

662 What anatomical abnormalities are associated with testicular torsion?

663 How is a patient with suspected testicular torsion treated?

664 Classify testicular tumours.

665 How do we investigate a patient with a suspected testicular tumour?

666 How is orchidectomy performed for a testicular tumour?

667 Outline the use of radiotherapy and chemotherapy in the management of testicular tumours.

668 What is a hydrocele and what may be its cause?

669 How can hydroceles be treated?

670 Compare the fluid from a hydrocele, spermatocele and an epididymal cyst.

671 What is the significance of a varicocele and how may it be treated?

672 How can patients with impotence be treated?

673 What do we mean by undescended, maldescended and retractile testes?

674 Where might you find a testis if it is not palpable in the scrotum?

675 What problems are associated with undescended testes?

676 When and how should undescended testes be treated?

677 How should a male with infertility be investigated and can the infertile male be successfully treated?

678 What are phimosis and paraphimosis?

679 What are the causes of erectile dysfunction and how do we investigate it?

680 What information should be given to a patient prior to a vasectomy?

THE HEART, LUNGS AND THORACIC CONTENTS

681 How might someone fracture a rib and what problems might it cause?

682 What is 'flail chest' and how do you manage it in the first hour after trauma?

683 What is pneumothorax?
   What classification do you use?

684 What is tension pneumothorax and what would YOU do about it?

685 Three operations on the pleura are often confused: Pleurodesis, Pleurectomy, Decortication.
   Can you say what is involved in each?

686 What is surgical emphysema and what does it imply?

687 What happens if there is a bullet or knife wound through the chest wall?

688 A mobile chest X-ray is a standard part of the assessment of an injured patient but you may be more familiar with films taken in X-ray departments.
   Are there any differences in their interpretation?

689 What are the general indications and principles involved in the use of chest drains in trauma patients?

690 A victim of a sudden deceleration accident appears to have a wide mediastinum on X-ray.
What would you do?

691 What would you consider in a patient presenting with haemoptysis?

692 What are the clinical and radiological features of a pleural effusion?

693 What are the more important causes of pleural effusion?

694 How does lung cancer typically present?

695 How is the diagnosis of lung cancer confirmed?

696 Where do we look for evidence of spread in bronchial carcinoma?
How does that influence management?

697 Mediastinal lymphadenopathy may be seen on plain X-ray or chest CT.
What is the differential diagnosis?

698 What are the indications for thymectomy?

699 What is an empyema and how is it treated?

700 What is bronchopleural fistula?

701 Which groups are most at risk from pulmonary tuberculosis these days?

702 A patient presents with back pain and X-rays show a collapsed thoracic vertebra.
What might be the cause?

703 In the first edition of this book we asked about fungal lung infections and our answer at that time did not include AIDS!
In what other groups of patients would you suspect fungal pulmonary infection?

704 Who are likely to inhale foreign bodies and with what consequences?

705 What do you know about mesothelioma?

706 When would you suspect a diagnosis of

endocarditis and how would you confirm your suspicions?

Does surgery have any role in its treatment?

707 What is an aneurysm and what types occur in the thoracic aorta?

708 What is aortic dissection and what are its lethal consequences?

709 What is the initial management of dissection of the aorta?

710 What are the neurological complications of aneurysms of the thoracic aorta?

711 Outline the possible consequences of the ductus arteriosus remaining open into adult life.

712 Explain the clinical and chest X-ray features of coarctation of the aorta.

713 What are the four features that give Fallot's tetralogy its name?

714 What is the cause of mitral stenosis and how can it be treated?

715 Give some of the long-term complications that all doctors should be aware of in patients who have undergone valve replacements.

716 How would you recognize aortic stenosis clinically?

717 What are the indications for coronary artery bypass grafting?

718 What patients with angina may gain prognostic benefit by having a coronary operation?

719 Doctors are not infrequently led off the track when patients with coronary artery disease do not complain of 'pain'.

What does 'angina pectoris' actually mean? Can you think of other diseases called 'angina'?

720 Some mechanical complications of myocardial infarction are referred for surgery.

What are they?

721 Can you give a numerical answer to the following questions?
  a) What is the risk of dying after a coronary artery bypass operation?
  b) What is the chance of complete relief of angina at a year after bypass surgery?
  c) What is the probability of being alive at 5 years?

NEUROSURGERY

722 A previously well 56-year-old woman has a grand mal seizure. Clinical examination and skull X-ray are normal.
  Is further investigation required?

723 A 45-year-old patient complains of severe headache, and neck stiffness is found on examination.
  What points in the history help determine the cause?

724 A 60-year-old man with recent weight loss of about 6 kg, develops difficulty in walking followed by difficulty with micturition.
  What is the most likely diagnosis?

725 In the above, what clinical signs would support this diagnosis?

726 Is it necessary to admit all patients with a skull fracture for observation?

727 A patient presents to the A&E department after sustaining a 'minor' head injury.
  What points in the *history* indicate the severity of the injury?

728 What neurological features are important in the assessment of head-injured patients?

729 What is the Glasgow Coma scale?
  Why was it developed?

730 Why is the pupil reaction to light important in head injury assessment?

731 How can limb weakness be detected in a comatose patient?

732 What radiological investigations are of most value in head injury?

733 What is the most frequently occurring type of traumatic intracranial haematoma?

734 What sites of skull fracture are associated with extradural haematoma formation?

735 Only one in two patients in coma after head injury has an intracranial haematoma.
What causes the depression of conscious level in the remainder?

736 What is the treatment of acute intracranial haematoma?

737 How do patients with chronic subdural haematoma present?

738 What operative treatment is required for chronic subdural haematoma?

739 Skull X-ray reveals a depressed fracture, underlying a deep laceration.
Is any treatment other than suture of the laceration required?

740 What are the clinical features of raised intracranial pressure?

741 Why should lumbar puncture be avoided in someone with suspected raised intracranial pressure?

742 If an intracranial tumour is suspected, what investigations should be carried out?

743 Does Magnetic Resonance Imaging (MRI) have any advantage over CT scanning when examining the brain?

744 What are the common types of malignant intracranial tumour?

745 An HIV-positive patient has an intracerebral mass on CT scanning.
What are the possible causes and what are the first steps in management?

746 Can intracranial meningiomas be removed completely at operation?
Does incomplete removal matter?

747 How does an acoustic neuroma present?

748 How may pituitary tumours be classified?

749 What neurological deficit may be produced by pituitary tumours?

750 What are the possible routes of approach for operative removal of pituitary tumours?

751 Is lumbar puncture still used to confirm subarachnoid haemorrhage?

752 A ruptured intracranial aneurysm is the commonest cause of subarachnoid haemorrhage.
What are the other possible causes?

753 When a third nerve palsy presents along with clinical features of subarachnoid haemorrhage, what is the likely cause?

754 What radiological investigations are required to identify the cause of a subarachnoid haemorrhage?

755 If the patient survives the initial bleed from a ruptured aneurysm, what complications may follow?

756 What are the risks of rebleeding from a berry aneurysm?

757 How can bleeding from an intracranial aneurysm be prevented?

758 How may arteriovenous malformations of the brain present?

759 What features on plain spinal X-rays would suggest that cord compression is due to metastatic tumour?

760 What benign lesions cause spinal cord compression?

761 What clinical features suggest disc protrusion at the L5/S1 level?

762 What is hydrocephalus, and what are its causes?

763 How is hydrocephalus managed?

764 Who was Harvey Cushing?

EAR, NOSE AND THROAT

765 What is a tympanogram and how does it help in the diagnosis of 'glue ear'?

766 Describe exactly how you would syringe the ear.

767 What is meant by so-called 'malignant' otitis externa?

768 A purulent discharge from the ear may occur with otitis media or externa.
How can you tell them apart?

769 What is 'glue ear'?
What are the causes?

770 Which organisms usually cause acute otitis media?

771 How could you distinguish between 'safe' and 'unsafe' chronic suppurative otitis media?

772 Long-standing chronic suppurative otitis media may lead to serious complications.
What are they?

773 What is otosclerosis and how does it present?

774 What are the characteristic features of Ménière's disease?

775 What is an acoustic neuroma?
How does it usually present to an ENT surgeon?

776 Does tinnitus, when it is the only symptom, merit further investigation?

777 What are the typical features of presbyacusis?
Does a hearing aid help?

778 What is the significance of cerebrospinal fluid running from the ear following a head injury?
What would you do about it?

779 How would you deal with a patient with a broken nose?

780 What are the common causes of nose bleeds?

781 How would you treat a patient with a nose bleed?

782 List some causes of a blocked nose.

783 What is the treatment for perennial allergic rhinitis?

784 What is submucous resection of the nasal septum?

785 Allergy to dust or grass pollen is a common cause of nasal symptoms.
What is the immunological mechanism involved?

786 How may sinusitis be distinguished from other causes of nasal symptoms?

787 How is sinusitis treated?

788 The prognosis for most patients with cancer of the nasal sinuses is poor.
Why?

789 What part do the tonsils and adenoids play in childhood obstructive sleep apnoea?
In principle how do you deal with this problem?

790 How can the nasopharynx be examined?

791 How does cancer of the nasopharynx present?

792 What are the common causes of an ulcer on the tongue?

793 What is meant by a globus sensation?
Is it an important complaint?

794 How would you diagnose a pharyngeal pouch?

795 What is post cricoid carcinoma and how is it treated?

796 If a GP sees a patient with a hoarse voice, when should he refer him for a specialist opinion?

797 How can listening to the pattern of noisy breathing help in localizing the level of the airway obstruction?

798 What is epiglottitis?

799 A hoarse, weak voice is sometimes due to unilateral vocal cord paralysis.
       What is the likely cause?

800 What is the treatment for laryngeal cancer?

801 How would you deal with a patient whose only complaint is a symptomless lump in the neck?

802 What are the indications for tracheostomy?

803 What are the most important points in the immediate postoperative management of tracheostomy patients?

THE EYES

804 What are the signs of dysthyroid eye disease and how may vision be lost in this condition?

805 How would you examine a patient who complained of a 'floating speck' in the vision of one eye?

806 What are the possible causes of unilateral proptosis in a woman of 45?

807 What is the ocular complication of oxygen therapy in premature infants?
       How may it be avoided?

808 How may a cerebral tumour present to an ophthalmologist?

809 How may sarcoid affect the eye?

810 How does conjunctivitis differ from iritis in its symptoms and signs?

811 What are the ocular complications of herpes zoster affecting the trigeminal nerve?

812 What is a chalazion?

813 What is a dendritic ulcer?
      What are the right and wrong ways of treating it?

814 How may fluorescein be utilized in the diagnosis and investigation of eye disease?

815 What might make you think that someone had suffered a corneal abrasion?
      How would you deal with it?

816 What causes of a subconjunctival haemorrhage do you know?

817 What sort of treatment should a chemical burn (acid or alkali) to the eye receive?

818 Is conjunctival pigmentation an important finding?

819 What are the symptoms and signs of acute glaucoma?

820 What are the ocular complications of steroid therapy?

821 The mother of a 3-month-old child says that one of its eyes has been watering since birth.
      What is the differential diagnosis?

822 Describe the symptoms and signs of chronic simple glaucoma.

823 How does Chloroquine affect the eye and how may its effects be monitored?

824 Do you know how the drugs used in the management of acute glaucoma act to reduce intra-ocular pressure?

825 What circumstances may lead a casualty officer to suspect the presence of an intra-ocular foreign body and how may the diagnosis be confirmed?

826 Do you know any diseases which are associated with cataract formation?

827 What is meant by pseudophakia and why is it important?

828 When should cataract extraction be considered?

829 What are the symptoms of optic neuritis?

830 Describe the pupil responses to light in a patient with a left optic neuritis.

831 How may papilloedema be recognized?

832 What sorts of diabetic retinopathy do you know?

833 Can diabetic retinopathy be treated?

834 What symptoms might you expect from someone with choroiditis?

835 How may a choroidal melanoma present?

836 What is night blindness and what may it signify?

837 What are the causes of sudden loss of vision in a quiet eye?

838 What is amblyopia?

839 How may drugs vary the pupil size?

840 What are the indications for squint surgery?

841 How many lasers would be used in the treatment of ophthalmic disease?

842 What are the causes of a white pupil in a child?

ORTHOPAEDICS AND FRACTURES

Fractures: general

843 What is the difference between a simple and a

compound fracture and why is the distinction an important one?

844   When can a fracture be described as 'pathological'?
     Give some examples of pathological fractures.

845   What causes a stress fracture?

846   Describe the treatment of a compound fracture of the tibia in the first 6 hours after the injury.

847   What is the principal danger of applying plaster of Paris to a fresh fracture?
     How can this danger be avoided?

848   What indications do you know for internal fixations of fractures?

849   What are the advantages of external fixation of a fracture?

850   What is callus and what is its function?

851   How should fractures around the growth plate be classified and what is the clinical relevance of the classification?

852   Describe the clinical features of the fat embolism and ARDS syndrome following fractures.

853   What factors may cause delayed or non-union of a fracture?

854   What is acute compartment syndrome?
     What are its clinical features and treatment?

855   What are the degrees of peripheral nerve damage?

856   What is a 'greenstick' fracture?

Orthopaedics: general

857   What is the commonest organism responsible for osteomyelitis in children and how does it reach the bone?

858   How would you diagnose acute osteomyelitis in a child?

859 How should acute osteomyelitis be treated?

860 Why is chronic osteomyelitis so difficult to cure?

861 Why would you be concerned about the presence of metal or cement in the region of a bony infection?

862 How likely is it that a total hip replacement will become infected?
  What can be done to minimize this risk?

863 What special hazards are there in the surgical treatment of rheumatoid arthritis?

864 What is meant by the term débridement?

865 What is the classic deformity of the metacarpo-phalangeal joints in rheumatoid arthritis?

866 Describe the clinical progression of ankylosing spondylitis.
  Has surgery anything to offer patients with this condition?

867 Explain the difference between osteoporosis and osteomalacia.

868 What are the main causes of osteoporosis?

869 Describe the principal features of Paget's disease of the bone.

870 What are the clinical features of achondroplasia?

871 What musculoskeletal problems are encountered by a severe haemophiliac?

872 What is the commonest malignant tumour in bone?

873 Which group of patients is most at risk from osteosarcoma and what sites are most likely to develop this tumour?

874 Describe the investigations of a young adult with suspected osteosarcoma of the distal femur.

875 What is osteotomy and why may it be performed?

876 What is hemiarthroplasty and what is its most common application?

877 How long would you advise a patient that a hip replacement is likely to last?

878 What materials are commonly used in artificial joint replacements?

879 What are the common causes of failure of total hip replacement?

Orthopaedics: regional

The hip and femur

880 Explain how to measure true and apparent leg length.
   What is the usual cause of apparent shortening?

881 What is the Trendelenburg test?
   When may it be positive?

882 How do you measure fixed flexion deformity at the hip?

883 Explain why the blood supply to the head of the femur is in danger when injury occurs.

884 What structures contribute significantly to the stability of the hip joint?

885 How would you recognize clinically a fracture of the neck of the femur and why is there such a high mortality?

886 Intracapsular fractures of the neck of the femur often require replacement of the femoral head with a prosthesis.
   Why?

887 Why is posterior dislocation of the hip quite easily missed?

888 Describe a central dislocation of the hip.

889 When and how should congenital dislocation of the hip (CDH) be diagnosed?

890 Why is early diagnosis of CDH so important?

891 What risk factors do you know that increase the likelihood of a child's having CDH?

892 What is known of the underlying pathological process in Perthes' disease?

893 What are the likely problems that may arise around the hip joint in a child with cerebral palsy?

894 What symptoms would you expect from a child with a gradual slip of an upper femoral epiphysis?

895 What is the crucial investigation needed to make the diagnosis of slipped upper femoral epiphysis?

896 What are the possible causes of non-traumatic avascular necrosis of the head of the femur?

897 Describe the main contra-indications to total hip replacement.

898 How would you recognize a septic arthritis of the hip?

899 Describe the radiological appearances of osteo-arthritis of the hip.

900 Assuming that other major injuries have been excluded, what is the emergency treatment of a fractured shaft of the femur?

901 How should a fracture of the shaft of the femur be immobilized in the first 24 hours after injury?

The knee and lower leg

902 What are the functions of the menisci?

903 What is the normal angle of the femur on the tibia?

904 What is meant by a 'locked' knee and what are the usual causes?

905 How do you test for medial or lateral collateral ligament laxity?

906 What changes would you expect in the rest of the limb after any derangement of the knee?

907 How would you test an injured knee for anterior cruciate injury?

908 What radiological investigations are useful in assessing the injured knee?

909 Where is the commonest site for a meniscus to tear?

910 What is the likely course of events in the years following meniscectomy?

911 What investigations other than radiology are useful in assessing an injured knee?

912 What is osteochondritis dissecans of the knee and how does it present?

913 What do we mean by an unstable patella and how can it be treated?

914 What is genu varum?
Why is this deformity likely to give trouble?

915 What are the indications for high tibial osteotomy?

916 What is the important difference between a displaced and an undisplaced fracture of the patella?

917 What pathological process occurs in Osgood-Schlatter's disease?

918 Describe the ideal below knee amputation stump.

The ankle and foot

919 What surgical treatment is available for post-traumatic osteo-arthritis of the ankle?

920 What damage is done in the common 'sprained ankle'?

921 Why is it important to get anatomical reduction in fractures involving the ankle joint?

922 What is the difference between a bunion and hallux valgus?

923 What is hallux rigidus?

924 What is metatarsalgia?

925 What is the other name for club-foot?
    Describe the deformity.

926 Do flat feet commonly cause symptoms?

The spine

927 What plain X-ray films are taken in assessment of a neck injury?

928 Describe the place of MRI scanning in investigation of spinal disorders.

929 Outline the structure of an intervertebral disc.

930 A surprising degree of structural scoliosis may be missed on inspection of the back.
    What is the best method of demonstrating the deformity?

931 What is the significance of limitation of straight leg raising?

932 What physical signs would you look for in a patient with spondylolisthesis?

933 How should an unstable cervical spine be stabilized?

934 Where may a psoas abscess become palpable?
    What is the other major physical sign in this condition?

935 What symptoms are typical of spinal stenosis?

936 What can be done to prevent osteoporotic crush fractures of the spine?

937 All patients who have been hit on the head and concussed should have a radiograph of the cervical spine.

Where are serious injuries most commonly missed?

938 How are the majority of disc prolapses treated?

939 When is prolapsed lumbar intervertebral disc a surgical emergency?

940 What is the difference between 'laminectomy' and 'disc excision'?

941 Define spondylolisthesis, spondylolysis and spondylosis.

942 What can be done surgically for a spondylolisthesis of L5 on S1?

943 In developed countries, what is the commonest and most disabling form of scoliosis?

944 How should a patient with a suspected unstable injury of the thoracolumbar spine be nursed?

945 Why is it important that a patient with rheumatoid arthritis should have a neck X-ray before having an operation?

946 What is the usual treatment for an unstable injury of the cervical spine?

947 What were the main causes of death in patients with spinal cord injuries before the development of special centres for treatment?

The shoulder and arm

948 What are the clinical features of anterior dislocation of the shoulder?

949 What proportion of abduction of the shoulder is scapulothoracic and what proportion takes place at the glenohumeral joint?

950 What structures form the rotator cuff and what is its function?

951 Describe the course of the circumflex nerve. Why is this clinically important?

952 What views may be obtained in addition to the plain PA and lateral films when investigating the shoulder joint?

953 Why is posterior dislocation of the shoulder easily missed?

954 How do you reduce an anterior dislocation of the shoulder?

955 Explain the mechanism behind recurrent dislocation of the shoulder.
    What can be done surgically to treat it?

956 How would you treat a fractured clavicle in a young adult?

957 Sir Robert Peel, a Prime Minister in the nineteenth century and founder member of the Metropolitan Police, died of a fractured clavicle.
    Why did this kill him?

958 Which injuries of the upper limb require treatment with a collar-and-cuff sling rather than a long arm sling?

959 What is a 'frozen shoulder' in pathological terms?

960 Describe the painful arc syndrome.

961 What is the rotator cuff of the shoulder?
    Describe its function.

962 Describes a Colles' fracture.

963 How would you treat a Colles' fracture in an old lady?

964 Describe a Monteggia fracture-dislocation.

965 What is the principal danger of supracondylar fracture of the humerus in children?

The hand

966 How can you test the function of the deep and superficial flexor tendons to the fingers?

967 What is the usual sensory innervation of the hand?

968 What signs would you expect in a hand with chronic loss of median innervation?

969 What would you expect to find in a hand without ulnar innervation?

970 What is the only small muscle of the hand consistently innervated by the median nerve and how do you test it?

971 What is the main deficit if the radial nerve is divided above the elbow?

972 What types of grip do you know?

973 What is the blood supply of the scaphoid bone?

974 What is trigger finger?

975 The hand can get stiff very easily when injured. What can be done to avoid the oedema that leads to stiffness?

976 Which is more important to the function of the hand, muscle power or sensation?

977 Describe the diagnosis and treatment of a fractured scaphoid.

978 How can stable fractures of the phalanges be treated?

979 What is Bennett's fracture of the thumb?

980 What is often described as 'no man's land' in flexor tendon injuries?

981 What should a casualty officer do if he suspects a cut flexor tendon at the level of the proximal phalanx?

982 Why are infections liable to cause a great deal of damage to a hand?

983 What is the correct treatment if pus is suspected in a hand?

984   What is 'mallet' finger and how is it treated?

985   Describe a grease-gun injury to the hand.

986   What is the significance of a human bite injury over the metacarpophalangeal joint?

987   What are the symptoms and signs of carpal tunnel syndrome?

988   What is de Quervain's syndrome?

989   What is the clinical picture in Dupuytren's disease of the hand?

990   What is a ganglion?

WHAT IS . . . ?

991   What is a cyst?

992   What is a fistula?

993   What is a sinus?

994   What is an ulcer?

995   What is a carbuncle?

996   What is an empyema?

997   What is a cystic hygroma?

998   What is Courvoisier's Law?

999   What is Sister Marie-Joseph's nodule?

1000   Who was Gazornenplat?

2
Answers

'ON THE SPOT'

1   From the story and findings one can assume a
    major intra-abdominal event has given rise to
    peritonitis. While considering the differential
    diagnosis, I would put up a drip and arrange
    investigations before proceeding to appropriate
    treatment. The differential diagnosis is primarily
    between a perforated peptic ulcer and acute
    pancreatitis. Investigations required are full blood
    count, urea and electrolytes, serum amylase,
    'group and save' serum, erect and supine abdom-
    inal films, erect chest X-ray, and an ECG. In
    the absence of free gas on the X-ray, an amyl-
    ase over 1000 would suggest pancreatitis. If
    free gas is noted, however, or if the amylase level
    is non-diagnostic, operation is indicated.

2   Blood dripping from the nose or mouth is a
    certain sign of postoperative haemorrhage. If no
    blood is visible, excessive swallowing is suggestive
    that bleeding is continuing and the breathing may
    be noisy as the blood bubbles in the pharynx.
    Swallowed blood is very irritant to the stomach
    and a sudden vomit of fresh blood is an indication
    of significant haemorrhage. Later, there will be
    signs of shock with tachycardia, hypotension,
    pallor, sweating and restlessness. By this time,
    there is a serious threat to life.

3   In view of the recent cardiac history, this clinical
    picture is highly suggestive of mesenteric in-
    farction due to embolism of a mural thrombus
    formed on the infarcted myocardium. Other coin-
    cidental abdominal emergencies are possible, but
    much less likely.

4   The diagnosis of temporal arteritis should be sus-
    pected and this may be supported by a grossly
    raised ESR. Urgent temporal artery biopsy
    should be performed although therapy should not
    necessarily be delayed until the result is available.

Treatment consists of high doses of prednisolone in order to control the arteritis rapidly and to prevent contralateral ophthalmic artery occlusion which would result in total blindness.

5 Very little. A penny will pass through the alimentary tract of a 2-year-old without difficulty. The mother should be strongly reassured, but perhaps told to watch out for the coin in the child's stool. It can be expected to have passed by the sixth day.

6 If leaking aortic aneurysm is strongly suspected but unconfirmed, rapid preparations should be made for laparotomy, including the cross-match of 10 units of blood, at the same time as carrying out quickly several important investigations. An ECG should be done to exclude myocardial infarction, although the pain would be unusual for this diagnosis. Chest X-ray and abdominal films will allow a search for aortic calcification which may delineate an aneurysm and help to exclude other diagnoses. Abdominal ultrasound and CT scanning are also useful in the confirmation of an aneurysm if the patient's condition permits. Finally, a serum amylase should be done quickly to exclude pancreatitis. If a non-surgical cause of the presentation is not found then laparotomy should be performed with urgency.

7 He presents the clinical picture of Boerhaave's syndrome, and has suffered a rupture of the thoracic oesophagus, due to very high intra-oesophageal pressure caused by vomiting. The surgeon will arrange a chest X-ray to confirm rupture into the pleura, as is usual, and perhaps place a chest drain to relieve any cardiorespiratory embarrassment produced by the leak. The most important step is preparation for urgent thoracotomy to clean out the affected pleural cavity, débride the oesophageal tear, and lay open the mediastinal pleura to minimize chemical and bacterial mediastinitis. Two large chest drains will be inserted prior to closure. Broad spectrum antibiotics will be prescribed, and a feeding gastrostomy or jejunostomy made, so that the oesophagus is temporarily bypassed.

8 The first priority is to establish a cause for the confusion. The wound should be examined

together with the chest and abdomen. A chest X-ray should be arranged simultaneously with estimation of haemoglobin, urea and electrolytes and blood gases. Hypoxia and fluid/electrolyte disturbance are common causes of such confusion as is sepsis, which can occur without a pyrexia. The first priority is to treat the cause but the patient will require reassurance and good nursing. Sedation with analgesics, chlorpromazine or benzodiazepines should be a last resort as they may exacerbate the underlying condition.

9   The most likely causes of haematemesis in this young alcoholic are oesophageal varices and peptic ulcer, while others include erosive gastritis and a Mallory-Weiss tear. Management depends to a large extent on precise diagnosis, so, when resuscitation has been carried out, upper GI endoscopy is required to make the differential diagnosis.

10   The story suggests that the patient has renal colic, so early management includes symptomatic relief, and examination and investigation to establish the diagnosis and define the cause. He should be given adequate analgesia, always bearing in mind the possibility that the patient may be a pethidine addict in search of a 'fix'. A history of previous episodes, recent trauma or the symptoms of disordered calcium metabolism should be sought. The urine should be inspected visually, tested for blood and protein, sent for culture, and sieved for stones. An IVU is carried out soon after admission and blood taken for calcium estimation.

11   The clinical picture suggests two main possibilities, both causing diaphragmatic irritation — these are a subphrenic abscess and left lower lobe pneumonia. After physical examination, a chest X-ray is taken to look for signs of these lesions. However, this may not be conclusive as pneumonic changes can develop secondary to subphrenic abscess, and an elevated diaphragm can occur with pulmonary collapse and consolidation. Therefore further investigations are required, usually ultrasonography or X-ray screening of the diaphragm for paradoxical movement.

12   The first priority would be to resuscitate the patient by giving 24% oxygen, inserting an intravenous cannula, commencing an intravenous infusion and sending off blood for culture, full blood count, urea and electrolytes and blood gas estimation. Whilst waiting for the portable X-ray and ECG machines to come, a full clinical assessment should be made. The most likely diagnosis is an anastomotic leak with Gram-negative septicaemia. Alternative explanations are a pulmonary embolus or myocardial infarction. If a pulmonary embolism is seriously considered, a VQ scan should be arranged.

13   The story of vomiting so much blood is usually exaggerated by a frightened patient or relative. Nevertheless, is sounds as though a significant bleed has occurred, and it must be assessed with urgency. If the patient shows obvious signs of haemorrhage, it is best to put up a drip, arrange baseline blood tests and cross-match 2 to 4 litres of blood at the outset. Next, a history and examination may reveal use of ulcerogenic drugs in view of his arthritis, in which case a peptic ulcer or gastric erosions should be suspected. In this age group carcinoma of the stomach is also a possibility. After adequate resuscitation, upper GI endoscopy should be performed to define the source of the bleed. Further management involves careful monitoring and blood replacement; gastric erosions usually respond to conservative therapy, while if the diagnosis is peptic ulcer, surgery will be required for major continuing or repeated haemorrhage.

14   No. A major intraperitoneal haemorrhage is in progress and requires urgent laparotomy if exsanguination is to be avoided. Careful anaesthesia should not influence the outcome of the head injury. If the patient simultaneously shows evidence of an intracranial haemorrhage, then exploration of the head and abdomen can be performed simultaneously.

15   The most likely cause of this patient's breathlessness is a pneumothorax which has progressively enlarged and is now under tension. The original minor accident may have caused one or more rib fractures with injury to the lung, leading to pro-

gressive accumulation of air; the presence of surgical emphysema would confirm the suspicion. Increased resonance and reduced or absent breath sounds on the side of the lesion will be found and deviation of the trachea and displacement of the apex beat would support the diagnosis of tension. Whenever possible, a chest X-ray should be seen before an attempt is made to treat pneumothorax, but in an emergency the tension should be relieved by insertion of an IV cannula between the ribs. If the diagnosis is correct, air will rush out with an audible hiss and the patient's distress will be relieved rapidly.

16 The history strongly suggests recurrent transient ischaemic episodes, which are usually due to small emboli shed from atheromatous ulcers in the extracranial carotid arteries. Petit mal fits are the other possibility. If there is a history or signs of atheromatous disease, especially if a carotid bruit is present, the doctor must refer the patient urgently for a vascular opinion, as early carotid surgery may prevent a dense stroke or even death.

17 All the features of this story suggest a diagnosis of intussusception, a condition seen in weaning babies in which one part of the bowel, usually the distal ileum, telescopes into the lumen distal to it, possibly due to the action of peristalsis on hypertrophied mucosal lymphoid tissue. The diagnosis can often be made on the history and examination, but X-rays, including barium enema, may be required to confirm it. Examination may reveal a mass, usually in the upper abdomen. Rectal examination occasionally detects the head of the intussusception in the rectum; on withdrawal of the finger bloody mucus will be found on the glove in most cases. Plain X-ray will show small bowel obstruction, while a barium enema will produce the typical 'coiled spring' pattern as the contrast spreads between the head of the intussusception and the surrounding small bowel wall.

18 He has almost certainly developed a pseudocyst of the pancreas. In this condition the lesser sac fills with an exudate consisting mainly of pancreatic secretion, surrounded by a layer of acute inflammatory tissue. The best way to confirm the

diagnosis is by ultrasonography; lateral barium studies will show a mass pushing the stomach forwards.

19   This man has almost certainly suffered a pelvic fracture which has caused injury to his membranous urethra. Catheterization, especially by someone like me, is liable to induce further damage to the urethra, so I would leave his further urological assessment to the urologists. While they were coming, I would examine the patient carefully to exclude any other important injuries.

20   Having checked that the patient does not require immediate resuscitation, the cause of the bleed should be sought. Sometimes such a bleed is due simply to piles, but a large haemorrhage in a patient in whom there is blood in the rectum without an obvious anal lesion is most likely to be bleeding from diverticular disease or angiodysplasia. In both conditions the blood is usually dark. Haemorrhage stops spontaneously in at least 80%, so that bed rest and blood replacement are all that are required in the short term. If haemorrhage continues, selective angiography is the best way to site the bleeding — barium studies and colonoscopy are usually unhelpful. Radiographic detection of one of these lesions in a patient who continues to bleed is an indication for emergency resection.

21   The circulation must be maintained and the blood oxygenated with the absolute minimum of delay if there is to be any chance of success. The sequence of priorities is important. Look at the patient quickly checking for carotid pulse or heart sounds and for any obvious, reversible cause such as an obstructed airway. A call for help is issued as soon as a genuine emergency is confirmed, which should take only a second or two, and cardiac massage started with adequate force and rate. After 4 or 5 seconds give the first couple of breaths of mouth-to-mouth respiration. Maintain massage and ventilation as long as you are on your own. As help arrives, delegate and share tasks according to the relative experience of the personnel available. Record the sequence of events as accurately as possible after the crisis is over if you were first on the scene.

22 The most likely cause of this clinical picture is carcinoma of the oesophagus or cardia, although there are other possibilities; dysphagia for solids but not liquids suggests a mechanical hold-up, so a benign stricture could be present, but this is unlikely without a history of heartburn due to a hiatus hernia. Occasionally this picture can result from compression of the oesophagus by a mediastinal mass, such as advanced bronchial carcinoma. Investigation will include a barium swallow to confirm a mechanical lesion and show its outline (a carcinoma will show as an irregular stricture of variable length, perhaps with shouldering), and endoscopy which will allow direct visualization and biopsy.

23 The patient has developed a 'burst abdomen'. When the sutures in the deeper layers gave way, the wound discharge was misinterpreted as a wound infection. You should ask the nurses to apply warm moist packs to the bowel loops and to prepare the patient for theatre. He will require resuturing of his abdominal wound under general anaesthetic.

24 All the clinical features point towards a diagnosis of ischaemic colitis. This condition is commonest in people with pre-existing atheromatous disease. Pathologically, it consists of an ischaemic lesion, usually involving the splenic flexure of the colon, affecting the mucosa primarily. In most cases the symptoms resolve on conservative measures.

25 The patient has probably developed a 'false aneurysm' due to detachment of the graft from the arterial wall. The diagnosis can be confirmed by an ultrasound scan and arteriography.

26 The unconscious patient who has been the subject of major trauma needs careful but rapid assessment of systems in a particular order of priority. Great care must be taken if there is any suspicion of a spinal injury particularly in the cervical region. Immediately the airway must be checked and cleared; difficulty with ventilation, either due to upper airway damage or chest injury, may require the passage of an endotracheal tube, especially as hypoxia causes brain swelling, exacerbating the head injury. At the same time major

external haemorrhage must be stopped. Major thoracic injuries, producing pneumo- or haemothorax, must be recognized and dealt with next. The abdomen is then examined, looking for evidence of 'run-over' injury and intraperitoneal haemorrhage, using lavage if uncertain. All the above types of injury carry an immediate threat to life. What remains are the medium-term problems, including assessment of the head injury — perhaps including the giving of dexamethasone to reduce cerebral oedema — a check for pelvic and urological injuries, and finally limb injuries.

27 It sounds very much as though he has developed gas gangrene, either due to simple inoculation of the organism into a dirty wound, or as an endogenous infection due to perforation of the rectum by the spike. There are four things to do to save his life: first, he must be started on large doses of penicillin to try to confine the clostridial infection; second, an EUA is necessary to decide if the bowel has been damaged — pre-operative X-rays will also help — and if this has occurred a proximal colostomy is required; third, the buttock wound must be carefully débrided, to remove dead and dirty tissue; finally, treatment in a hyperbaric oxygen chamber is required to eradicate the clostridial infection.

28 He is suffering from intermittent swelling of a submandibular salivary gland, probably due to a stone in Wharton's duct.

THE ACUTE ABDOMEN

General clinical features

29 The cardinal features of such a pain are its constancy, and the fact that it is made worse by movement. The constancy contrasts with the intermittent pain caused by the muscular contraction of an obstructed viscus. The movements which exacerbate this pain may include those due to breathing, coughing, yawning or movement of the whole body, as in turning over in bed — hence the patient tends to lie very still.

30 Patients commonly present in casualty with abdominal pain from urinary infections or stones in

the urinary tract. This may show up as an increased protein and blood content in the urine.
Less common findings are glycosuria in patients
with diabetic ketoacidosis, a raised bilirubin concentration in patients with acute cholecystitis and
a colour change from orange to port-wine colour
in patients with porphyria.

31 The diaphragm receives its nerve supply from the
same roots as the skin over the shoulder and so
pain in the shoulder may result from diaphragmatic irritation. Bleeding from a ruptured
spleen or ruptured ectopic pregnancy can irritate
the diaphragm. Bowel contents can track there
from a perforated viscus and this may be followed
by pus from intra-abdominal sepsis.

32 These are abdominal colic, distension, vomiting
and constipation. The precise order in which the
symptoms occur helps determine the anatomical
level of the obstruction.

33 While 'faecal' vomiting indicates the actual vomiting of faeces, the term 'faeculent' means that the
vomitus merely simulates faeces. Faeculent vomiting occurs in established small bowel obstruction — the vomitus becomes brown and offensive
due to the heavy overgrowth of bowel organisms.
This relatively common finding must be distinguished from the rare faecal vomiting which follows gastrocolic fistula due to benign peptic ulcer,
or cancer of the stomach or colon.

34 While guarding is a reliable sign of significant
intra-abdominal pathology, tenderness is less so.
The presence of tenderness is a subjective sign,
requiring palpation followed by the patient's interpretation of what it felt like. While intra-
abdominal lesions such as appendicitis and
cholecystitis will certainly induce tenderness, this
sign may also be found in patients with non-
specific 'tummy upsets' or even in the nervous
patient without demonstrable pathology. Guarding, on the other hand, is a more objective
physical sign. It is similarly demonstrated by
gentle abdominal palpation and is produced by a
sustained reflex increase in the resting tone of
the abdominal wall muscles, either locally or
generally, in response to parietal peritoneal
inflammation of whatever cause. It should be

carefully distinguished from the sudden increase in tone produced by the clumsy examining hand, confusingly known as 'voluntary guarding'.

35 An erect chest film and a supine abdominal film are usually requested on patients presenting with abdominal pain. The erect chest film will show gas under the diaphragm following an intra-abdominal perforation and the abdominal film will show distended loops of bowel if obstruction is present. Traditionally an erect abdominal film was also requested, but this rarely gives any additional information to that given by the other two films, hence radiologists have argued that it should be abandoned.

36 The most common and hence most important, conditions which can cause acute abdominal symptoms are pneumonia and cardiac disease, either failure or infarction. Another very important group are childhood acute viral illnesses. Pneumonia, especially involving the bases, can produce marked abdominal pain, with tenderness and guarding, while acute cardiac disease, perhaps due to hepatic engorgement, can cause a similar picture. Upper respiratory tract infections in children are sometimes accompanied, or even masked, by an abdominal syndrome mimicking appendicitis. Careful questioning will usually elicit the relevant non-abdominal symptoms. Other less common problems are raised by herpes zoster, diabetes and very rarely porphyria and syphilis.

37 Central back pain, usually accompanied by other characteristic symptoms and signs, is often present in cases of acute pancreatitis and in leaking aortic aneurysm. Central pain may also be present in those with an acute exacerbation of gastric or duodenal ulcer symptoms, in whom the ulcer is penetrating the posterior wall to involve the pancreas. Lateral back pain, particularly in the loin, may be due to renal or ureteric disease, usually a stone. Higher on the right, such pain may indicate acute cholecystitis or biliary colic.

38 We listen for bowel sounds. If these are absent then the patient may have peritonitis leading to a paralytic ileus; if increased and tinkling the patient may have bowel obstruction.

Appendicitis

39   In pathological terms, appendicitis usually develops secondary to obstruction of the appendiceal lumen, leading to infection of the pent-up
mucus. In children this may be due simply to
hypertrophy of a lymphoid follicle in the wall of
the appendix, while in adults a faecalith is the
more common cause. Unusually, appendicitis
follows luminal obstruction due to caecal carcinoma, Crohn's disease or the presence of fruit
seeds or intestinal worms.

40   The first symptom in this condition is usually
central abdominal pain. Soon afterwards anorexia
and malaise develop, while the pain moves within
a few hours to the right iliac fossa, where it is constant and worse with movement. Vomiting may
occur in unspectacular amounts, while the bowel
habit may be unchanged, constipated or some-
what loose. On examination, the patient usually
looks listless and may be flushed. The tongue is
dirty and the temperature usually raised no higher
than 38°C. Unless perforation has occurred,
breathing movements of the abdomen are present
but palpation reveals tenderness, guarding and
rebound tenderness. Rovsing's sign (RIF pain following the rebound test in the LIF) is a reliable
sign. Rectal examination is required only if the
diagnosis is not obvious after abdominal examination; pelvic appendicitis is best confirmed this
way.

41   The appendix, like the rest of the bowel, is innervated solely by the autonomic system. Intestinal
autonomic pain is poorly localized and felt in the
midline. As with the rest of the mid-gut,
appendiceal pain occurs around the umbilicus. As
the condition progresses, the inflammatory process spreads through the wall of the appendix to
involve the parietal peritoneum. This excites the
somatic nerves supplying the abdominal wall,
enabling the patient to locate the pathology accurately to the right iliac fossa.

42   This point lies at the junction of the lateral third
and medial two-thirds of a line joining the right
anterior superior iliac spine and the umbilicus. It
has three important uses: anatomical, clinical and
operative. Anatomically it roughly indicates the

surface marking of the base of the appendix, clinically it is usually the site of maximal tenderness in appendicitis, while at operation, it marks the midpoint of the classical McBurney's incision for appendicectomy.

43 The appendix is examined to confirm the diagnosis of appendicitis. Sometimes the inflammation may have come from outside the appendix in which case the cause must be sought. Rarely Crohn's disease or caecal carcinoma may be present. Incidental findings include carcinoid tumours and threadworms.

44 The most likely explanation is that the patient has developed an appendix mass. This usually develops in a case not treated within 4 or 5 days of the onset of symptoms. The omentum has become wrapped around the appendix, producing a phlegmon, or simple inflammatory mass. Operation is avoided, as appendicectomy would be difficult and hazardous due to the danger of damaging the bowel around the mass. However, should the temperature begin to swing, suggesting an abscess had developed, or if signs of spreading peritonitis appear, surgery is required. Less likely, but very important causes of an RIF mass in a patient with suspected appendicitis are Crohn's disease, or a caecal carcinoma which is obstructing the appendix.

45 The accuracy of diagnosing appendicitis is about 80% so diagnostic laparoscopy could save patients from unnecessary appendicectomy. More recently the appendix has been successfully removed via the laparoscope but this is still an experimental technique.

46 Metronidazole is routinely given before operation, as a suppository or intravenously on induction, to reduce the risk of infection with non-sporing anaerobes such as *Bacteroides*. In addition cephalosporins or aminoglycosides are given as prophylaxis against enterobacteria such as *E. Coli*.

Biliary disease

47 The illness begins with worsening epigastric and

right subcostal pain, which becomes severe, constant and worse during inspiration. The pain may radiate to the right scapular region. Nausea and vomiting are variable. On examination the patient, usually female and often obese, will have a moderate pyrexia. Occasionally a fleeting jaundice will be noted. Tenderness and guarding will be found mainly in the right subcostal region. Murphy's sign (reflex inhibition of inspiration when the examining hand is pressed under the costal margin) is often present.

48 Yes. The remarkable feature was the severity of the pain. The patient had developed right upper quadrant pain a few hours before; the pain was agonizing and constant unlike intestinal colic. She retched violently several times. Although she was in a cold sweat, the temperature was normal. The gall-bladder was palpable and fairly tender. The pain was greatly relieved by an injection of pethidine and did not return when the pethidine wore off.

49 Yes. Ultrasonography and HIDA-radio-isotope scanning can both be used. Ultrasonography can confirm the presence of gall-stones, demonstrate the thickened wall of the gall-bladder and determine whether it is distended. HIDA-scanning involves injecting an isotope-labelled substance which is rapidly excreted in the bile. In acute cholecystitis, the obstructed gall-bladder will not admit the labelled bile and therefore will not be visualized on a scan. Clinical diagnosis alone is wrong in 10 to 15% of cases of acute cholecystitis, so these tests are particularly useful if surgery is practised routinely in the acute phase.

50 Most surgeons treat acute cholecystitis conservatively. The aim is to 'rest' the gall-bladder in the knowledge that the episode will settle within a week without complications in 85% of patients. As gall-bladder contraction is stimulated by cholecystokinin, released from the duodenum when chyme enters it, gall-bladder 'rest' requires cessation of oral intake and hence intravenous fluids.

51 This is a rather controversial question. Some surgeons believe that all patients with this diagnosis should undergo cholecystectomy at the next elec-

tive operating list, arguing that this halves the period of hospitalization and that urgent surgery does not increase mortality, morbidity or difficulty of operation. Most surgeons have yet to adopt this policy; their indications are therefore much more limited, involving only the 15% of patients who go on to develop empyema or gangrene of the gall-bladder, or biliary peritonitis, all diagnosed by careful clinical monitoring during conservative management.

52 After taking blood cultures the patient should have a drip and be started on intravenous antibiotics such as aminoglycosides or a cephalosporin. The diagnosis is most likely to be a stone in the common bile duct as the patient has the triad of symptoms described by Charcot. This could be confirmed by an ultrasound examination. An elderly frail patient could have the stone removed at ERCP by sphincterotomy and Dormia basket extraction. If there were residual stones in the gall-bladder, a later cholecystectomy might be indicated.

53 Gall-stone ileus. In this condition, gas enters the biliary tree via a cholecystenteric fistula — usually into the duodenum — caused by the erosion into the bowel of a large gall-stone. The stone then passes down the gut to impact, producing obstruction. Another possibility is that the cholecystenteric fistula is iatrogenic, performed to relieve obstructive jaundice. This should be ascertained from the history, especially if a scar is found. The obstruction may then simply be due to postoperative adhesions. However, one must not be distracted by the interesting X-ray from checking the hernial orifices.

Perforated peptic ulcer

54 Perforated duodenal ulcers are fairly uniform in appearance — almost always the perforation is circular, about 3–5 mm in diameter and looks so neat that it might have been made with a ticket-punch. Occasionally a piece of undigested food will be seen impacted in the perforation. The duodenal wall around the defect is usually stiff and friable due to oedema. The site of perforation

in over 90% of cases is the middle of the anterior wall of the first part of the duodenum.

55   Duodenal ulcers in the anterior wall of the duodenum erode through into the peritoneal cavity and so cause peritonitis. Those in the posterior wall erode backwards into the gastroduodenal artery and so cause haemorrhage.

56   The erect chest X-ray. The cardinal radiological sign is free gas under the diaphragm and this can be missed on the erect abdominal film. The reason for this is that the X-ray exposure necessary to penetrate the abdomen is greater than that for the chest. Thus, even though the diaphragm may be included in the erect abdominal film, it may not be visible due to the high X-ray exposure, so that subphrenic gas will appear in continuity with the lung and hence be missed. The chest X-ray, however, exposed so as to show fine lung detail, will demonstrate the diaphragm with gas below and lung above. Nevertheless in 30% of perforations gas is not present under the diaphragm.

57   Yes, always a serum amylase and often an ECG. All the symptoms and signs of perforated ulcer can, and often do, occur in acute pancreatitis. Myocardial infarction can sometimes present as an 'abdominal catastrophe', so this possibility must be excluded if doubt exists. Basal pneumonia will already have been excluded by the routine erect chest X-ray. Having taken these precautions, laparotomy is mandatory despite the lack of free gas on X-ray as the latter is not seen in 30% of perforations, while other conditions which can mimic perforated ulcer, such as mesenteric infarction and leaking aneurysm, all require operative management.

58   The usual operations are simple oversew for duodenal ulcer and partial gastrectomy for gastric ulcer. Oversew in duodenal ulcer is most surgeons' choice as it is quick and safe, the ulcer is never malignant and 25% will never have any further ulcer symptoms. However, some surgeons believe more definitive ulcer surgery, usually vagotomy, should be performed, especially in those with a history of dyspepsia. Simple oversew

is never enough in gastric ulcer — 10% of these are malignant and the ulcer is often large and ragged, making closure impossible or unsafe. Most surgeons therefore, would do a Billroth 1 gastrectomy, while others would excise the ulcer to exclude malignancy and perform a vagotomy.

59   There is no doubt that surgery offers the best chance for survival if the patient can withstand the operation. Therefore, the assistance and advice of a senior anaesthetist and a physician where indicated should be urgently sought with the aim of improving the general condition sufficiently to allow surgery. With non-operative management several outcomes are possible. The ulcer may seal and the condition gradually settle, the free gastric fluid may lead to a localized abscess such as subphrenic, or septicaemia and death may supervene. Management should therefore include meticulous nasogastric suction to minimize leakage, careful fluid balance, broad spectrum antibiotics to cover the expected septicaemia and a watch for abscess formation. The patient is best nursed semi-erect so that any abscess formation is pelvic rather than subphrenic. This position will also aid breathing in these sick patients.

60   Corticosteroids, aspirin, phenylbutazone and most of the more recent anti-inflammatory analgesics are not only ulcerogenic, but also increase the risk of perforation in pre-existing peptic ulcers.

Complications of diverticular disease

61   Diverticulosis refers merely to the presence of diverticula and is present in 30% of the population over the age of 60, most of whom are symptomless. Diverticulitis on the other hand, is the illness which develops when a segment of colon, usually the sigmoid, involved in diverticulosis, becomes the seat of an acute inflammatory process.

62   This is a nickname for acute diverticulitis. It refers to the similarity in the progression of symptoms and signs between these two conditions. Thus, in diverticulitis, the patient

often describes a vague lower abdominal pain which later localizes in the left iliac fossa and on examination there is peritonism in the same area.

63 The diagnosis is usually fairly straightforward, with a story of localizing LIF pain, pyrexia, localized peritonism and perhaps, a tender mass. In females a tubo-ovarian infection should be excluded and in both sexes evidence of perforation sought and the possibility of carcinoma remembered. Initially, treatment is conservative, comprising starvation, IV fluids, antibiotics (a cephalosporin or gentamicin, with metronidazole) and analgesia. Usually the condition settles over 4 to 5 days, although in a few, clinical signs and X-rays will suggest abscess formation or spreading peritonitis due to perforation, requiring urgent surgery. Following uneventful recovery from an uncomplicated episode a high fibre diet should be started and a barium enema, perhaps with colonoscopy, should be arranged to exclude a carcinoma. Repeated episodes of diverticulitis or failure to exclude carcinoma are indications for elective sigmoid colectomy.

64 The clinical picture presented by a pericolic abscess is similar to that of uncomplicated acute diverticulitis. The differences which suggest this diagnosis are the temperature which begins to swing, and the presence of a tender mass, although this can occur without abscess formation. Later cases may develop overlying erythema. Clinical suspicion should be followed by ultrasonography. Once diagnosed, the abscess should be drained; this can usually be done by scanguided intubation or direct incision in the LIF, though sometimes formal laparotomy is needed to be sure of the diagnosis. Elective resection is usually performed at a later date.

65 The attacks suggest recurrent urinary tract infections. These may simply be due to bladder outflow obstruction secondary to an enlarged prostate predisposing to infection. But more rarely the diverticular disease may have produced a fistula into the bladder (a vesicocolic fistula) and the bowel contents may be infecting the urine.

66 The Hartmann's procedure involves resection of the sigmoid colon with formation of an end left

iliac fossa colostomy and oversewing of the rectal stump. It is popular in perforated diverticular disease as it removes the involved segment while avoiding the more complicated procedure of primary anastomosis. Some surgeons advocate the latter, with or without a protective proximal stoma.

67 Poor. Untreated this is uniformly fatal, due to septicaemia and renal failure. Even after surgery, especially if primary resection has not been possible, about 50 to 60% of patients with faecal peritonitis will die. This is due to the usually advanced age and frequent intercurrent cardiorespiratory disease, coupled with the septic and renal complications of faecal peritonitis.

Acute pancreatitis

68 In this country, about 60% of cases occur in patients with gall-stones and there is strong evidence for a causal relationship. A further 20% are due to alcoholism, while the remainder are due to a myriad of factors, including steroid therapy, trauma (sometimes iatrogenic), hyperparathyroidism, mumps and several others. A few cases remain idiopathic. In countries where alcoholism is more prevalent, acute pancreatitis is correspondingly more common.

69 Although the presentation is rather variable, the usual picture is one of steadily increasing abdominal pain, peritonitic in nature, which may be epigastric or generalized. There is often a 'band-like' upper abdominal pain radiating to the back. The patient is usually nauseated and often vomits. On examination there is commonly a mild pyrexia, tachycardia and slight cyanosis. There is epigastric or generalized peritonism, sometimes to the extent of board-like rigidity. Bowel sounds may be diminished or absent.

70 Clinical suspicion will lead to taking of a blood sample to measure the serum amylase; if this is more than 1000 Somogyi units, the diagnosis is confirmed. If the serum amylase is less than 1000, pancreatitis is still possible, but other conditions such as perforated peptic ulcer and acute cholecystitis must be actively considered. Some-

times, with an amylase below 1000 and a high suspicion of perforated ulcer, laparotomy will be necessary, leading to macroscopic diagnosis of pancreatitis.

71   Initial management comprises the treatment of shock and the recognition and treatment of any respiratory, renal and metabolic complications as early as possible. Treatment of shock entails fluid, protein and sometimes blood replacement, preferably with regular central venous pressure monitoring. Respiratory complications are frequent and should be anticipated by blood gas analysis on admission and regularly thereafter. If the Po_2 falls below 70 mmHg, oxygen should be given. Further deterioration may require ventilation or tracheostomy. Renal failure, transient in the majority, occurs in up to 20%. Bladder catheterization and hourly urine measurements are mandatory from the outset. Oliguria should be actively treated by ensuring an adequate circulating volume followed by administration of diuretics. Other complications such as hypocalcaemia and clotting disorders must also be watched for. Pain relief is usually adequate with pethidine; peritoneal lavage is also useful in pain relief. Recently, some surgeons have advocated surgical drainage of the necrotic pancreas in progressively deteriorating cases. There is no proven place for the use of the antitryptic agent, Trasylol, or for glucagon.

72   The size of the rise in the serum amylase is a poor prognostic indicator. Ranson in New York has identified criteria which identify the high risk patient — these include old age, a large rise in the blood sugar concentration, a high white cell count, deranged liver function tests, a high blood urea and a large base deficit. Similarly a poor prognosis is associated with a marked fall in serum calcium and arterial oxygen concentration.

Vascular conditions

73   Mesenteric embolism usually occurs in the superior mesenteric artery. The involved bowel, therefore, will be part or all of the mid-gut, the precise extent depending on how distally in the arterial system the embolus lodges. Thus, if it

comes to rest in the trunk, all the bowel from the distal duodenum to the mid-transverse colon will be at risk of infarction. Mesenteric infarction is an extremely serious condition, with a high mortality. 'Treatability' depends on the amount of bowel involved and the age and general condition of the patient. If at laparotomy the bowel is dead from duodenum to splenic flexure, it is probably best to close the abdomen. If, however, even 30 cm of small bowel is alive, then in the younger patient resection should be performed. However, subsequent nutrition may require permanent intravenous feeding, a formidable prospect, available in only a few units in this country.

74   A history of rectal bleeding following on from non-specific but severe abdominal pain may suggest mesenteric infarction. On examination the patient may have atrial fibrillation and a temperature. Blood tests may show a high serum potassium and raised white count. X-rays may show the thumb print pattern, or linear gas shadows within the bowel wall. Absence of bowel gas (the 'ground glass abdomen') is another characteristic X-ray feature.

75   The patient with a leaking aortic aneurysm is usually suffering from severe abdominal and back pain. The patient is usually hypotensive and may present with loss of consciousness due to the hypotension. The condition may therefore mimic a head injury or a heart attack. If the leak is small and posterior the patient may be thought to have renal colic. It may be mistaken for other intra-abdominal emergencies including perforated peptic ulcer, diverticular disease or pancreatitis.

76   No. The diagnosis having been made on the basis of the age, frequently associated cardiovascular disease elsewhere, the history of sudden onset of bloody diarrhoea, localized left abdominal tenderness and diagnostic X-ray changes, the patient is treated conservatively with a good prospect of recovery within a few days. In a few the presentation is more dramatic, with evidence of peritonitis on admission, while in others this may develop after beginning conservative therapy. These patients require laparotomy and resection urgently. A few who recover on a conservative regimen later

develop troublesome symptoms due to stricture — these also require surgery.

Gynaecological conditions

77 Acute salpingitis, ruptured pyosalpinx, ovulatory bleeding, twisted ovarian cyst and ectopic pregnancy. Less commonly, a twisted or degenerating fibroid or a bleeding endometrioma can cause confusion.

78 The patient may be simply ill or in extremis, depending on whether the Fallopian tube has ruptured. If the bleeding is still contained in an intact tube, then the patient will typically give a history of one or two missed periods, with recent onset of hypogastric pain — usually colicky — and variable vaginal bleeding. On examination, she will look uncomfortable and there will be suprapubic tenderness, perhaps more on one side and pelvic examination should reveal a tender fornical mass. A much more dramatic and potentially fatal picture is seen after the tube has burst, releasing the tamponade, to allow free peritoneal haemorrhage. The patient will tell of a sudden onset of severe peritonitic pain, perhaps radiating to the shoulders. She will be pale, with a thready pulse. The abdomen may be distended and will be tender with guarding. Pelvic examination will be very uncomfortable and the fornical mass should be palpable. This picture should lead to rapid diagnosis and life-saving surgery, preferably by a gynaecologist.

79 These two conditions may be difficult to distinguish; sometimes laparoscopy or even 'grid-iron' laparotomy is required in very doubtful cases. Distinction is usually possible, however, on clinical grounds. Salpingitis is not usually heralded by peri-umbilical pain and salpingitic pain is normally suprapubic, often bilateral or even confined to the left side. A history of vaginal discharge should always be sought. On examination the site of tenderness in each disease corresponds to the site of pain; pelvic examination is always necessary in young women, looking for vaginal discharge, cervical pain on manipulation and tender adnexae. A confident diagnosis of salpingitis will save the patient an operation.

Intestinal obstruction

80 In most cases, the cause will be found to be either an obstructed groin hernia or postoperative adhesions.

81 Intestinal obstruction disturbs the normal circulation of fluid between the blood and the bowel lumen. The 8 litres of fluid secreted in the upper alimentary tract each day are normally mostly reabsorbed in the distal small bowel. In distal obstruction, not only does this absorption stop, but active secretion into the bowel occurs. Thus large volumes of fluid are sequestered in the bowel, leading to clinical dehydration even before vomiting begins.

82 It means literally what it says. It occurs in patients with intestinal obstruction — as the bowel progressively distends with fluid, it begins to empty itself into the stomach leading to vomiting.

83 This is a particularly dangerous form of obstruction in which a loop of bowel is effectively obstructed at both ends and is best exemplified by the obstructing annular colonic carcinoma. Normally the ileocaecal valve prevents reflux of colonic content into the ileum; in large bowel obstruction, ileocaecal continence prevents retrograde transmission of pressure into the small bowel. The closed loop of colon becomes grossly distended and the high luminal pressure causes the occlusion of vessels in the bowel wall, leading to early perforation, usually in the caecum. Closed-loop obstruction can be diagnosed on X-ray and is an indication for urgent laparotomy. Luckily, the ileocaecal valve often fails to prevent reflux in large bowel obstruction, so that in such cases, the progression to caecal perforation is very unusual. Volvulus is another form of closed-loop obstruction.

84 This is essentially a clinical syndrome produced by incomplete intestinal obstruction. The patient complains of abdominal discomfort, perhaps with colic, and sometimes vomiting. The most important clinical feature is the continuance of bowel action, usually diarrhoea. On examination the abdomen may be modestly distended and the bowel sounds obstructive. Radiology will show dis-

tended loops with fluid levels. Patients may present having been in this stage for days, even a few weeks. Subacute obstruction is perhaps most commonly seen in slowly progressive conditions such as Crohn's disease or peritoneal metastatic carcinoma, but it can occur in colorectal cancer or postoperative adhesions. The place of surgery depends on the underlying pathology.

85   On admission, an estimate must be made of the abnormal fluid losses already suffered. This is done by assessing the clinical state — vital signs, the state of the tongue, tissue elasticity — together with the length of history and frequency of vomiting. Clinical dehydration is not detectable until about $2\frac{1}{2}$ litres have been lost in the average 70 kg man, while obvious dehydration will suggest a $4\frac{1}{2}$ litres deficit. The moribund patient may well be 7 litres in deficit. As a rule of thumb, all the fluid can be assumed to have been equivalent to normal saline containing 20 mmol of potassium per litre. Fluid therapy in the first 24 hours will comprise the normal maintenance requirement, that is approximately 3 litres of fluid, including 140 mEq sodium and 40 mmol potassium, plus the estimated abnormal losses to date.

86   In 1 litre of normal saline there are 153 mmol each of sodium and chloride. In fact this solution, otherwise known as physiological saline, is not 'normal' in the chemical sense, nor quite isotonic.

87   This is a solution containing 131 mmol of sodium, 5 mmol of potassium, 4 mmol of calcium, 111 mmol of chloride and 29 mmol of lactate per litre. It was introduced as a mixture containing similar electrolyte concentrations to plasma.

88   There are two main features, the position of bowel loops and the mucosal pattern visible in the distended bowel. As a general rule, the large bowel will occupy the periphery of the abdomen though the transverse and sigmoid segments may lie centrally, especially when distended. Small bowel lies centrally though it can appear to occupy the whole abdomen when distended. Mucosal pattern is a more useful pointer. Small bowel has a characteristic appearance — the mucosal folds, or valvulae conniventes, lie in regular sequence in the distended bowel, produc-

ing either multiple transverse bands or a series of ellipses. The haustra of the large bowel on the other hand, appear as more widely spaced ingressions only partially crossing the lumen. Knowing which parts of the bowel are distended helps decide the level of the obstruction and hence a plan for management. Distended small bowel alone, perhaps with a history of previous abdominal surgery and no evidence of external hernia, strongly suggests adhesion obstruction, which may be treated conservatively at first if the history is short, and there is no evidence of strangulation. Distended large bowel, indicating large bowel obstruction, strongly suggests that surgery should be performed after adequate resuscitation, as all the most likely causes are best remedied by operation.

89 Full blood count, assessment of patient's blood group, and urea and electrolytes. Although estimation of dehydration is mainly a clinical decision, the haemoglobin and blood urea help in this estimation. The electrolytes begin to change late in the natural history, so are a poor parameter of electrolyte depletion, but serve as a guide to progress on treatment. The white blood cell count is important when considering the possibility of strangulation. However, while a high white count is very worrying, a low count by no means excludes this complication.

90 You might suspect that the patient had a paralytic ileus rather than a mechanical obstruction to the passage of bowel contents. The diagnosis would be confirmed by a history of painless abdominal distension and on examination the patient would often have absent or diminished bowel sounds. The plain abdominal X-ray usually shows generalized gaseous distension of the bowel, including the rectum. A paralytic ileus is often associated with a low serum potassium.

91 No. Although usually a sign of intestinal obstruction, in very thin people, especially if old or emaciated, the abdominal wall can be so thin that normal peristalsis may be visible.

92 Metabolic acidosis, developing as a result of dehydration and under-perfusion of body tissues, particularly the splanchnic circulation. Acidosis can

be particularly severe in the presence of strangulated bowel. A precise assessment is made by arterial pH measurement and blood gas analysis. The mainstays of correction are adequate resuscitation and the removal of dead tissue. It is uncommon to need to give bicarbonate, but if the patient is shocked or develops cardiac arrhythmias, an initial dose of 80 mmol of sodium bicarbonate is a sensible step.

93 The few useful signs all involve the presence of gas in abnormal positions. First, free gas in the peritoneal cavity indicates perforation and strangulation or ischaemic perforation due to stretching of bowel wall are the likely causes. The other signs are more subtle; the presence of a thin line of gas a few millimetres lateral to the luminal gas shadow and parallel to its edge indicates gas in the bowel wall and is a sure sign of dead bowel. Finally, retroperitoneal gas or bubbles around the bulge of a groin hernia, also indicate dead bowel. All these signs are urgent indications for operation.

94 Plain abdominal films are important in diagnosis, but barium enema offers definitive diagnosis and, in some cases, a mode of treatment. The plain films will confirm intestinal obstruction and also the characteristic absence of gas in the right abdomen. Barium enema will demonstrate an ileocolic intussusception — the classical 'coil-spring' appearance produced as the barium spreads between the advancing intussusception and the bowel wall, is usually seen. So long as the history is no longer than 24 hours and there is no clinical suspicion of gangrene, the hydrostatic pressure transmitted by barium enema can be used to reduce an intussusception.

95 Any gynaecological procedure, or appendicectomy.

96 As a general rule, acute intestinal obstruction is an indication for surgery after initial resuscitation. However, adhesion obstruction, especially if recurrent, is best treated conservatively at first, unless there is a long history or any worry at all about strangulation. The advantages of conservatism are that many cases will settle on nasogastric suction and IV fluids and that further surgery,

while relieving the obstruction, may well make the adhesions worse, inviting future problems. If a conservative approach is used a very careful watch for deterioration is imperative and anyway, if no improvement is seen within say 36 hours, then surgery is necessary.

97 Colostomies and ileostomies are fashioned in patients with bowel obstruction when it proves impossible or unsafe to relieve the obstruction and at the same time join up the bowel again. For example following resection of diverticular disease in the sigmoid colon it may be unsafe to anastomose the colon and a colostomy may be fashioned (the Hartmann procedure). Some patients with obstruction are considered too ill for a bowel resection and they may simply have a 'defunctioning stoma' made to relieve the obstruction.

98 Yes — 'bolus' and 'Stammer's loop' obstructions. Bolus obstruction, due to the impaction of a mass of undigested food in the distal small bowel, is especially liable after gastrectomy as access to the small bowel is so rapid. Avoidance of pithy fruit and careful mastication should be impressed upon gastrectomy patients. Stammer's loop obstruction occurs when a variable length of small bowel becomes twisted around the afferent and efferent loops of the antecolic gastrojejunal anastomosis. This usually occurs within 3 weeks of gastrectomy and presents with the features of high small bowel obstruction. Early surgery is mandatory once the diagnosis is made.

99 The anaesthetist will be worried that a patient with obstruction is dehydrated and will want to check the recent urinary output, the patient's pulse and blood pressure and the patient's serum electrolytes. Correction usually involves an intravenous infusion with normal saline and added potassium chloride. Bowel obstruction will often dilate the stomach so that the anaesthetist will want a chest X-ray to exclude pre-operative inhalation of gastric contents, a nasogastric tube to empty the stomach and during induction cricoid pressure applied by an assistant to prevent regurgitation into the bronchial tree.

100 Certain clinical pointers do exist, but none is completely reliable. Strangulation sometimes

produces a peritonitic, constant pain super-imposed on the colic. On examination, the development of tenderness, especially if a mass is palpable, is a worrying sign as are pyrexia and tachycardia over 100 per minute. Hypotension, especially with pyrexia, is more common if strangulation has occurred.

101 The site of pain and the timing of onset of vomiting and absolute constipation differ. Small bowel obstruction usually causes colicky pain in the epigastrium or peri-umbilical area, while large bowel colic is likely to be hypogastric. Vomiting begins soon after the onset of pain in high small bowel obstruction, but for progressively more distal obstruction the vomiting occurs later, so that in distal large bowel obstruction this symptom may not appear at all. Constipation on the other hand has the opposite relationship — it is noticed almost immediately in sigmoid obstruction, while normal bowel activity may continue for 24 hours in high small bowel obstruction.

102 Carcinoma.

103 Spurious means inappropriate or misleading. Spurious diarrhoea is a symptom of incipient large bowel obstruction. The classical story in spurious diarrhoea is one of a recurring cycle of several days of constipation, followed by an episode of loose, even incontinent bowel actions. The diarrhoea occurs because the only motion able to creep past the obstruction is liquid stool. It is important to differentiate this pattern of bowel habit from infective diarrhoea and colitis, in which diarrhoea is usually continual.

104 Yes, several. First, as the most common cause of large bowel obstruction is carcinoma, it is extremely unlikely that the obstruction will settle spontaneously. Therefore a prolonged period of non-operative treatment is liable to lead to fluid balance problems, and the various complications related to bed rest, such as DVT. Another important possibility is the development of closed-loop obstruction with the risk of perforation. Therefore, in a case of large bowel obstruction, once adequate resuscitation has been performed, it is best to proceed to surgery without undue delay.

105 This a form of large bowel obstruction due to twisting of the sigmoid colon around the axis of its mesocolon. The sigmoid colon thus forms a closed loop, and may become massively distended, filling the abdomen. At presentation the patient may give a history of similar previous episodes which may have settled spontaneously. This condition seems to be more common amongst patients in mental institutions.

106 After adequate resuscitation, the patient requires an operation, the prime aim of which is to relieve the obstruction. In inexperienced hands, the emergency operation should be a laparotomy to confirm the diagnosis and to fashion a defunctioning transverse colostomy. Definitive resection and colostomy closure follow as one or two stages in the ensuing weeks. For more experienced surgeons the emergency procedure will usually involve the resection of the carcinoma. There is an increased risk of anastomotic breakdown in this setting as the bowel is distended and usually loaded with faeces, so the surgeon will usually fashion a proximal temporary colostomy to protect the anastomosis.

107 Dilated bowel can be seen when there is a paralytic ileus present. This is most commonly seen in the immediate postoperative period after abdominal surgery or in the presence of peritonitis. Rarer causes include hypokalaemia, uraemia and following trauma to the lumbar spine. In severe ulcerative colitis, the colon may dilate in a condition known as toxic megacolon.

108 This is the term applied by surgeons to a very small primary colonic tumour sometimes found at laparotomy for obstruction. The lesion is so small that at first sight the obstruction looks as though it could simply be due to ligature — or string — tied tightly around the colon.

Abdominal trauma

109 The first priority is to safeguard the airway, check for breathing, commence an intravenous infusion, cross-match blood and assess the conscious level. The patient will probably require an urgent CT

scan and elective ventilation. As soon as possible the patient should have peritoneal lavage performed to exclude significant intra-abdominal damage from a crushing injury because the head injury will mask the usual signs of intra-abdominal injury.

110 In most patients there will be a history of blunt abdominal or lower chest trauma within the previous few hours, though in some it may have occurred several days previously. They will complain of variably severe abdominal pain, worse on movement and often referred to the left shoulder. On examination, there will be pallor and signs of hypovolaemia. Abdominal examination will reveal local or generalized tenderness and diminished bowel sounds.

111 Surgeons may try to preserve the spleen if it is injured to reduce the risk of the patient subsequently developing overwhelming sepsis. This is a particular problem in young children. If the spleen is too badly damaged to be preserved, then it is sometimes possible to implant splenic tissue and all patients should have pneumococcal vaccination postoperatively.

112 As the nerves supplying the abdominal wall are usually T8 to T12, trauma to the chest wall can bruise or damage these nerves as they pass along the line of the ribs. This can produce reflex spasm of the abdominal wall musculature, mimicking the picture produced by intra-abdominal injury, even when all is well within the peritoneum.

113 Any penetrating wound up to the level of the sixth rib, or roughly the level of the nipples, may have entered the abdomen, as the domes of the diaphragm reach up to this level.

114 The organs most likely to be injured by a seat-belt are those that are relatively fixed in position within the abdomen, so that they cannot slip out of the way when squeezed by the belt, and especially those lying in front of the spinal column. Thus the organs most at risk are the stomach and bladder (especially when either is full), the duodenum, pancreas and small bowel with its mesentery.

115   While stab wounds to the abdomen cause visceral injury in only 30% of cases, bullet wounds from a hand-gun almost always produce some visceral damage, while velocity missiles always produce major destruction along the bullet track. A knife blade often deflects movable viscera as it enters the abdomen, though relatively fixed structures are more vulnerable; low-velocity bullets, as from a hand-gun, dissipate their kinetic energy rapidly as they penetrate and may be deflected by important structures. High-velocity bullets however, have enormous energy, causing explosive destruction of tissue several centimetres each side of the track, often causing fatal injury.

116   A stab wound involving the anterior wall of the stomach may well have penetrated the posterior wall also, perhaps even injuring the pancreas. Therefore these structures must always be inspected by formal opening of the lesser sac — otherwise these life-threatening injuries may be missed.

117   This is a collection of blood enclosed within the capsule of the spleen developing as a result of blunt trauma. Its significance is that, although the patient may have minimal symptoms and signs of splenic injury, the haematoma can rupture several days after the initial trauma, accompanied by further haemorrhage from the damaged parenchyma and this can be serious or even fatal. If such an injury is suspected the patient should be observed in hospital and subjected to radio-isotope scanning of the spleen, which may demonstrate the haematoma as a 'cold' defect in the splenic image.

118   Severe blunt trauma to the abdomen can cause a rupture of the diaphragm due to the sudden rise in intra-abdominal pressure — abdominal organs may then pass into the chest, causing a major impairment to vital capacity and ventilatory efficiency. The left diaphgram is damaged more often than the right, which is protected by the liver; stomach, colon and small bowel can all pass up into the chest.

119   The most sensitive investigation to check for intraperitoneal haemorrhage is peritoneal lavage; the bladder is emptied with a urinary catheter and

a peritoneal dialysis catheter is inserted below the umbilicus aiming towards the pelvis. A litre of normal saline is introduced and then siphoned out; a red cell count of >100 000/mm^3 is 'positive'. Contraindications are the urgent need for laparotomy on clinical grounds whatever the outcome of the paracentesis, pregnancy and previous lower abdominal surgery.

120 There are no pathognomonic radiological signs of ruptured spleen, but useful pointers are: posterior fractures of the left lower ribs, which lie behind the spleen; rightward shift of the gastric air bubble; fluid between coils of intestine; and elevation of the left diaphragm.

121 This test is unreliable and hence can lead to bad decisions. Moreover, it is evidence of visceral damage rather than merely of peritoneal penetration which is important, so probing of the wound need never be considered.

122 Chest X-ray will show loss of the normally clear line of the diaphragm, usually on the left, with partial collapse of the lung and perhaps a fluid level within a displaced abdominal viscus. Free gas, due to pneumothorax or ruptured viscus, may also be seen.

123 Bullet wounds to the abdomen always require laparotomy due to the high likelihood of visceral damage. Blunt trauma and stab wounds require exploration only when careful initial or subsequent clinical and radiological examination provide any evidence suggesting visceral injury.

124 This group of patients will include those with blunt trauma or stab wounds in whom there is no evidence of visceral damage on admission. They require careful monitoring, watching for evidence of intraperitoneal haemorrhage or leakage from a hollow viscus. Having taken blood for crossmatching and base line investigations, the vital signs are monitored hourly to begin with, and the abdomen examined frequently for signs of peritoneal irritation. Any change suggesting visceral damage should lead to operation. If all is stable at 48 hours the patient can usually be discharged, but if there is a possibility of intrahepatic or

intrasplenic injury, a longer watch should be kept,
and ultrasound or isotope scanning performed.

125 The patient with an abdominal knife wound
needs a general examination to exclude other injuries checking airway, breathing and cardiac output. An intravenous infusion should be started
and blood taken to assess haemoglobin concentration and to cross-match the patient in case of
further haemorrhage. Some surgeons follow a
policy of immediate surgery for all knife wounds
whilst others closely observe the patient, only operating for signs of intra-abdominal bleeding or
peritonitis. Other signs such as the presence of gas
under the diaphragm, omentum protruding from
the abdominal wound or probing of the wound
are no longer absolute indications for laparotomy.

126 Ampicillin, gentamycin and metronidazole; this
combination will cover the broad spectrum of organisms likely to be spilt from a lacerated large
bowel. Some surgeons might replace ampicillin
and gentamycin with a cephalosporin.

127 The surgeon will first try to decide whether the
external appearance of the liver reflects the internal damage — sometimes a small surface laceration hides an extensive intrahepatic haematoma
with major vessel damage and major devitaliza-
tion of liver tissue. If bleeding is occurring, he
may try to control it temporarily, while he assesses
the injury, by placing a non-crushing clamp on
the structures in the free edge of the lesser omentum — Pringle's manoeuvre. If the injury is considered local, bleeding is controlled and the liver
wound may be closed with sutures or omentum.
If the internal damage is more major, then either a
wedge resection to remove dead and bruised tissue or even a right hepatic lobectomy will be performed.

Water, electrolytes and nutrition

128   About 1200 ml of water is taken in by drinking.
      The water content of solid food contributes about
      a litre and a further 300 ml on average is gener-
      ated in the course of metabolism. The normal
      urine output is of the order of 1500 ml with about
      900 ml insensible loss from breathing and perspi-
      ration in a temperate climate, and about 100 ml
      lost in faeces.

129   Water is required to match the predicted losses, to
      correct a pre-existing deficit and to correct any
      additional losses during the 24 hours. The pre-
      dicted losses should allow 1500 ml for urine and
      1000 ml for insensible loss. Since the operation
      was routine it is likely that the patient left the op-
      erating theatre in balance, but it is likely that there
      will be some addition to be made for nasogastric
      aspirate or other drainage. A total allowance of 3
      litres is fairly typical.

130   There may be clinical evidence of water deficit or
      excess at the outset and a correction for this
      should be made in the fluid orders for the next
      period. All abnormal losses from fistulae, drains,
      diarrhoea and nasogastric aspiration must be
      accounted for and the fluid charts from the pre-
      vious 24 hours should contain this information.
      Increased insensible loss due to fever or
      tachypnoea should be allowed for. The urine
      output should be measured and if it is low the
      possibility of renal failure must be carefully
      considered before ordering extra fluid.

131   A typical intake of sodium is 75 to 100 mmol but
      it is highly variable from day to day and from one
      individual to another. The healthy kidney can
      conserve or excrete sodium over a very wide range
      by producing urine containing few millimoles or
      several hundred millimoles of sodium per day.

132 This is below the normal range which is about 135 to 145 mmol. This is rarely due to true sodium depletion but more commonly to an excess of circulating water, either infused as 5% dextrose, or the result of inappropriate ADH secretion. Apparent hyponatraemia can occur if there is an unusually large proportion of non-aqueous material in the serum sample, such as fat or protein.

133 A high serum sodium may be due to excessive infusion of sodium chloride, when there is usually oedema due to water retention. Alternatively, it can occur with water depletion; the hypernatraemia is unlikely to be gross except in diabetes insipidus, for instance with a basal skull fracture.

134 About 80 mmol of potassium per day is lost in the urine which accounts for virtually all the daily loss. The minimum urinary potassium loss is about 20 mmol/litre.

135 Abnormal losses from the gastro-intestinal tract over a long period can result in hypokalaemia. Examples are prolonged nasogastric aspiration, loss from fistulae, and diarrhoea in particular due to ulcerative colitis or villous tumours. Prolonged treatment with some diuretics can cause potassium depletion. Treatment of diabetic coma with insulin results in intracellular movement of potassium causing an acutely low serum potassium. Cardiac dysrhythmias, including ventricular fibrillation, may result. Lesser but more common consequences are general lethargy and muscular weakness.

136 Sometimes this is caused by a haemolysed sample so it is always worth checking if it does not fit the picture. There is a fear of cardiac arrest so it would be prudent to monitor the patient. The most likely cause is renal failure so check the urine output and other evidence of renal impairment. Meanwhile, once hyperkalaemia is confirmed, the quickest way to bring the potassium down temporarily is with a mixture of 25 g glucose and 10 units of insulin.

137 The aspirate is a mixture of gastric, pancreatic and small bowel secretions and bile and is likely to contain 100 to 150 mmol/litre of sodium and 5 to

10 mmol/litre of potassium. A replacement regimen of volume for volume normal saline with 10 mmol of potassium chloride added to each litre should be given in addition to other fluids. This should be modified in the light of the clinical progress and the results of serum electrolyte estimations. Electrolytes can also be measured in aliquots of the aspirate to confirm the initial estimates.

138   As a rule of thumb, replacement with normal saline with 10 mmol per litre of potassium chloride should be instigated. This should be added to the daily ration allowed for urinary and insensible loss. However, as this may require chronic management a day by day balance should be calculated, and the patient's clinical state assessed to ensure that the overall water balance is being maintained. Similarly measurements of electrolytes in the urine and in aliquots of the fistula fluid can be used to produce a balance sheet for the electrolytes. Measurement of serum electrolytes may only identify gross discrepancies because of the ability of the kidneys to correct for inappropriate fluid loss.

139   The main danger in infusing potassium chloride is that it is easy to produce a transient hyperkalaemia, which may cause cardiac arrest. The best way to prevent this is to avoid high concentrations of potassium and not to infuse more than 20 mmol per hour. Potassium can also produce ischaemic ulceration of the skin if allowed to run into the tissues.

140   About half the serum calcium is protein bound, about 45% is ionized and the remainder is present in solution but complexed with organic ions such as citrate.

141   Calcium is mobilized from bones in hyperparathyroidism and in malignant disease such as myelomatosis or advanced breast carcinoma. There may be increased absorption in vitamin D overdosage, sarcoid or milk alkali syndrome. Severe hypercalcaemia results in coma and anuria. Less severe, chronic hypercalcaemia causes calcification in the kidneys, constipation, vomiting and a generalized feeling of illness and depression.

142 Vomiting over a long period or nasogastric aspiration when the fluid is replaced with magnesium-free solutions can result in magnesium depletion. The loop diuretics can also have this effect.

143 Following surgery there is an expected catabolic period when the body's protein is used to provide energy. A patient who is already cachectic tolerates this poorly and may become acidotic with a rising urea. Healing and resistance to infection may be poor.

144 For the average adult an IV regime should contain 2000 to 3000 calories, a balanced supply of the essential amino acids to give 10 to 20 g of nitrogen, the essential fatty acids, vitamins and trace elements in addition to the usual ration of water and electrolytes. The calories can be supplied as glucose alone, adding insulin if required, or mixtures of ethanol, sorbitol and fat suspensions can also be used.

145 The biggest worry in intravenous feeding is infection on the central line. The patient can also be made hyperosmolar, hypoglycaemic or forced into lactic acidosis depending on which solution is used and how fast it is given. Because of these concerns, whenever possible we feed patients enterally, often through fine bore tubes and continuous flow rather than resorting to 'parenteral feeding'. Usually the intensive care unit or the gastroenterological team supervise feeding of such critically ill patients.

Management of the circulation

146 Shock is a term used to indicate failure of the circulatory system. The typical features are pallor, cold peripheries, sweating, tachycardia, oliguria and hypotension. The causes include loss of circulating volume due to acute haemorrhage; acute depletion of extracellular fluid due to conditions such as intestinal obstruction or burns; acute severe heart failure, when it is called cardiogenic shock; or sudden changes in the peripheral resistance or permeability as occurs in Gram-negative septicaemia.

147 The term hypovolaemia means that there is insufficient fluid in the vascular compartment to maintain an adequate circulation. In addition to evidence of poor circulation as witnessed by tachycardia, cool peripheries, small volume peripheral pulses, reduced urine output and eventually arterial hypotension there should also be evidence of reduced filling pressure to make the diagnosis — a low jugular venous pressure or, more reliably, a low central venous pressure indicates that there is hypovolaemic rather than cardiogenic shock. The volume mismatch is usually due to loss of intravascular volume but occasionally it is due to inappropriate dilatation of the vessels.

148 Blood, plasma protein fraction, dextran, gelatin, electrolyte and glucose solutions can all be used to expand the circulation. Electrolyte and glucose solutions are readily available and are, in relatively small volumes, fairly innocuous but they do not stay in the circulation and can produce salt or water overload if used to maintain circulating volume. The larger molecular weight solutions stay in the circulation longer but do not carry oxygen, and dextran may cause bleeding abnormalities. Blood loss if more than a litre is best replaced with blood. This may not be immediately available, needs cross-matching and may cause reactions.

149 The central venous pressure is a measure of the right atrial pressure and therefore of the filling pressure of the heart. It indicates the volume in the circulation, and it indicates when to continue and when to stop transfusion in a volume depleted patient. If, in spite of a central venous pressure of 10 to 15 cm, the circulation is still inadequate, there is an additional, probably cardiac cause.

150 In clinical examination of any injured or acutely ill patient, the first important assessment of the venous pressure is by clinical examination. The important diagnostic information is whether it is above or below normal. If there is a need to know the central pressure with more precision, or to monitor it continuously, the standard technique is by an internal jugular cannula with its tip in the

superior vena cava or right atrium. The most commonly used routes are internal jugular and subclavian veins, and relatively short catheters about 15 cm long can be introduced percutaneously in the neck or below the clavicle. Alternatively, longer lines can be threaded up from the arm. The catheter is connected to a giving set with a three-way tap in the system, so that the patient's venous circulation can form one side of a U-tube manometer and the pressure read off directly in centimetres of water, using the estimated position of the right atrium in the mid-chest as zero. This technique is usually performed by anaesthetists.

151 Oliguria is defined as an output of less than 500 ml per day. In the acute situation we monitor urine output more closely and prefer to see more than 0.5 ml/kg/hr. If the urine output is less than 20 ml per hour in 2 or more consecutive hours, some action should be taken.

152 The first step is to establish the underlying cause. Consider some pitfalls such as ruptured bladder or urethra (in the acutely injured patient) or a misplaced or blocked catheter in a patient already being monitored. Then the circulation should be assessed — is there adequate arterial pressure, peripheral low and central pressure? These should be restored towards normal with the aid of central venous pressure or Swan-Ganz measurement, if necessary.

153 Inadequate renal perfusion, septicaemia, jaundice, certain antibiotics including cephalosporins and aminoglycosides, haemoglobin from mismatched transfusions and myoglobin from crush injuries are factors that may contribute to the development of acute renal failure.

154 A diuretic challenge with frusemide may promote diuresis. Frusemide in doses of 250–500 mg IV may be given, and mannitol as 100 ml of 20% solution over 30 minutes. If a diuresis does not follow, begin fluid restriction and get expert help. Renal support by haemofiltration, peritoneal dialysis or haemodialysis may be needed whilst renal recovery is awaited.

155 Postoperative hypertension is hazardous because it increases the risk of bleeding at the operation site, can precipitate intracerebral bleeding and puts an increased work load on the left ventricle. The commonest cause is pain which should be assessed and relieved. Carbon dioxide retention due to respiratory difficulty should be dealt with if present. If severe hypertension persists, for example a diastolic pressure sustained at 120 mmHg, it could be treated with vasodilator drugs such as nitroprusside infusion and ideally this should be undertaken with the support of an intensive care unit.

156 Blood transfusion can cause circulatory problems, transfusion reactions or infection. The infusion of any solution which expands the blood volume can overload the circulation and cause heart failure and pulmonary oedema. If there is mismatch the reaction may include pyrexia, rash and hypotension. Haemolysis which releases haemoglobin into the circulation may result in acute renal failure if not promptly treated. Transfused blood can also be the source of infection, most notably with serum hepatitis, although this is now carefully screened.

157 Blood should be taken for the standard clotting tests and for a platelet count and the results discussed with the haematologist. The problem may be in the clotting factors, platelets, due to defibrination, or in the vessels themselves. The commonest cause is depletion of clotting factors and platelets due to replacement of surgical blood loss with old stored blood. This is treated with fresh frozen plasma, platelet concentrates or fresh blood. The prothrombin time is abnormal with liver disease and oral anticoagulants. The kaolin-cephalin time is abnormal in haemophilia. Clotting factor deficiencies of this kind can be corrected with a fresh frozen plasma from the transfusion laboratory. A platelet count below 20 000 per mm^3 can be responsible for a prolonged bleeding time but even if the count is normal, the activity may be reduced, as occurs with aspirin, and platelet concentrates may be necessary.

Postoperative complications

158 Infection is the most likely explanation and the wound, the chest and the bladder are possible sites. Deep infection related to the operation site must be considered. Another possibility is deep vein thrombosis, even in the absence of physical signs.

159 Bacteriological specimens should be obtained from the sputum and urine. Wound, faeces and blood cultures may also be indicated. A chest X-ray should be taken. A white cell count and differential should be done. Any clinical leads should be followed, such as ankle oedema or calf tenderness and appropriate special investigations arranged.

160 A swinging pyrexia suggests that there are episodes of bacteraemia and the most likely source is an abscess. The wound, pelvis or under the diaphragm are the most likely sites.

161 Haematoma, bacterial contamination, ischaemia, necrosis and foreign material contribute to wound infection. These all provide a culture medium which is kept around 37°C encouraging bacterial growth.

162 The anaerobic organisms play a large part in about 80% of infections complicating large bowel surgery and are not identified unless specific techniques are employed.

163 The first job is to drain the abscess. In many instances this is done surgically and a drain is left in the cavity to ensure that it does not reaccumulate. Inaccessible abscesses can be treated these days by aspiration through a wide bore needle but the general rules still apply. Antibiotics are a valuable adjunct to deal with associated bacteraemia and cellulitis but are not a routine part of the treatment of an abscess.

164 Sputum retention, patchy atelectasis and lobar consolidation may occur after major surgery. The secretions are thick after anaesthesia and pain reduces depth of ventilation and inhibits coughing; these contribute to the pulmonary complications.

The areas of atelectasis permit arteriovenous shunting and result in hypoxia.

165   The patient should be made as fit as possible pre-operatively by intensive physiotherapy and, if possible, surgery should be avoided in the winter months. Postoperative analgesic measures, local and systemic, help to preserve coughing but over-sedation must be avoided. Humidification helps to clear sputum.

166   Areas of lung which are not ventilated but still receive pulmonary blood flow represent areas of right to left shunt and cause arterial hypoxia. This can be recognized by the association of low Po_2 with a relatively low Pco_2 which happens because the hypoxia stimulates respiration and carbon dioxide is blown off to below normal levels.

167   Although chest infection can cause haemoptysis, pulmonary infarction due to thrombo-embolism is the probable diagnosis. If on the basis of the overall clinical picture this looks likely, urgent lower limb phlebography should be performed to confirm deep vein thrombosis so that treatment aimed at preventing further embolism may be started. The patient should then be heparinized, anticoagulation with warfarin initiated and local measures such as use of elasticated stockings used to discourage further thrombus formation. More detailed investigations to confirm pulmonary embolism such as ventilation/perfusion scans may follow but will not alter management in this particular clinical situation.

168   Virchow's triad comprises changes in vessel walls, changes in blood flow and changes in the composition of the blood; these three cause deep vein thrombosis. They are represented in the patient as local pressure on the calf vessels or pelvic vessels during surgery; venous stasis due to immobility; and increased number and adhesiveness of platelets.

169   While many are asymptomatic, the first clue may be a pulmonary embolus. The leg oedema, particularly unilateral, calf pain, tenderness and an unexplained low grade fever may all suggest deep vein thrombosis. The diagnosis is confirmed definitively by phlebography.

170   Anticoagulation should be commenced once the diagnosis of deep vein thrombosis has been confirmed by venography unless there are contra-indications such as continuing gastro-intestinal haemorrhage. Anticoagulation is commenced with heparin given as a bolus of 5000 units intravenously and continued at a rate of 1400 units per hour (or 17 500 units twice daily subcutaneously) with monitoring of the APTT (activated partial thromboplastin time) to give a level of about twice normal. Simultaneously warfarin is given at a dose of 10 mg/day for 2 days with the PTR (prothrombin time ratio) measured before treatment and on the third day. Heparin is then stopped and the dose of warfarin is adjusted to give a PTR of two to three times normal.

171   The clinical features depend on whether the embolism is massive, presenting with gross circulatory abnormalities, or smaller, presenting as pulmonary infarction. Massive pulmonary embolism causes sudden severe breathlessness associated with cyanosis, tachycardia, poor peripheral circulation and raised jugular venous pressure. All these features are due to sudden severe obstruction to blood flow in the pulmonary artery. Smaller emboli present as one or more episodes of haemoptysis and pleuritic pain associated with a rub. In addition, there may be signs of right ventricular obstruction. The diagnosis is confirmed by a ventilation/perfusion lung scan. The demonstration of areas of unperfused lung that are normal on the chest X-ray confirms and shows the distribution of emboli. A pulmonary angiogram is required if surgery is considered, though this is unusual.

172   Urgent heparinization is the treatment of choice in pulmonary embolism. In a small minority of patients who survive massive emboli but remain in a critical circulatory state, surgical removal, preferably on bypass, may be successful. Streptokinase infusion, particularly directly into the pulmonary artery, can succeed but is associated with troublesome complications.

173   Perioperative thrombus formation in the legs must be prevented. Subcutaneous calcium or sodium heparin given with the premedication and twice daily in the postoperative period has been

proven to reduce the risk. Low molecular weight heparin is simpler to administer and may have a lesser risk of bleeding complications, but its greater cost limits its widespread use. Local measures such as 'anti-embolism' stockings reduce venous stasis. The patient is kept mobile before and as soon as possible after surgery. Local calf pressure is avoided on the operating table and during the convalescence. Dehydration is avoided.

174 If there is evidence of poor peripheral circulation, poor urine output or arterial hypotension in spite of adequate filling pressures as judged from the jugular venous pulse or a CVP line, a myocardial cause should be suspected. A 12-lead ECG and a series of cardiac enzymes over the next 3 days will confirm the diagnosis of myocardial infarction.

175 Severe pain is a cause of tachycardia. If this has been excluded, the major causes are volume deficit and cardiopulmonary problems. The differential diagnosis depends basically on two things: what is the rhythm and what is the venous pressure? If the patient is in sinus rhythm and the venous pressure is low the circulation is underfilled. This should be rapidly corrected and any underlying cause such as haemorrhage dealt with. If there is a new abnormality in the rhythm such as atrial fibrillation, which may be precipitated by surgery, this should be treated appropriately. If there is sinus tachycardia with a high CVP this suggests a myocardial problem.

176 Primary haemorrhage occurs at the time of surgery. Reactionary haemorrhage occurs in the 24 hours following surgery and is generally due to missed primary haemorrhage, recovery from operative hypotension, or resolution of operative small vessel vasospasm. Secondary haemorrhage occurs about a week after surgery and most commonly happens with infected or open wounds, for example following haemorrhoidectomy or prostatectomy.

177 The blood loss must be replaced and the bleeding stopped. If cross-matched blood is available this should be given at a rate appropriate for the circulatory state and the rate of loss. Otherwise, the next most suitable fluid available should be given.

A member of the surgical team should make an urgent decision about re-exploration of the operation site, recognizing that the patient will stand further anaesthesia and surgery better if some time can be spent on resuscitation.

'LUMPS AND BUMPS'

178   On inspection the size, shape, smoothness or irregularity of its outline and its position in relation to anatomical landmarks may be noted. On palpation these findings can be confirmed and whether the lump is hard or soft, uniform or lobulated, hot or cold can be established. Its relationship to superficial and deep anatomical structures can be tested and the extent of tethering to these layers and the tests for fluctuance and transillumination performed.

179   To elicit fluctuance the lump is secured across a diameter between two fingers of one hand and gently pressed with the fingers of the other hand. Transmitted pressure to the securing fingers is interpreted as fluctance.

180   Tethering to the overlying skin or to deeper tissues may indicate invasion and therefore malignancy.

181   This is a useful trick to determine what layer a lump is in. If the muscles are tensed a superficial lump is more easily palpable while the borders of a deep lump become obscured.

182   A lump filled with clear fluid which is not too deeply situated will transmit light.

183   The lump would be red, hot, tense and tender.

184   A deep abscess should be suspected in a patient with spikes of fever, sometimes preceded by rigors and recurring every few hours. If it is sufficiently superficial a red, hot, tense and tender lump will usually be apparent. Abscesses require drainage.

185   Cellulitis is a spreading infection which tracks along subcutaneously or follows fascial planes. It is due to *Streptococcus* which produces an enzyme

called streptokinase which breaks down fibrin and prevents localization of the infection.

186 A boil is an infection originating in a hair follicle. There is a single abscess cavity just deep to the skin with surrounding inflammation. It discharges spontaneously through a central area of skin softening and then typically resolves quite promptly. A carbuncle is an area of infection in the subcutaneous tissues. There is more generalized necrosis and the pus is usually loculated in several smaller abscess cavities. The overlying skin may be lost as a slough leaving a necrotic area.

187 This description fits a lipoma, a lobulated, thinly encapsulated mass of fat which most commonly occurs superficially but can occur almost anywhere in the body. It is a benign lesion.

188 In Dercum's disease there are multiple, tender lipomata which are found particularly on the trunk.

189 A sebaceous cyst is found most commonly on the scalp. It appears hemispherical with smooth borders and a central punctum. It moves with the skin but is not fixed deeply. It is fluctuant but does not transilluminate.

190 Nobody knows. It is therefore difficult to evaluate the effectiveness of new treatments. They are due to a virus and it seems likely that variations in the body's immunological state may be responsible for the sometimes sudden and dramatic clearance of a crop of warts.

191 Keloid is overgrowth of skin in a scar. Scar hypertrophy is common but resolves within a few months, whereas true keloid progresses for a year or more and never fully resolves. It is more common in black skin.

192 'T' stands for tumour, 'N' for nodes and 'M' for metastases. T–0 indicates an undetected primary, while T–3 indicates a large or locally advanced primary. N–0 to N–3 indicate from no nodal involvement through anatomically more extensive lymphatic spread. M–0 means no detected distant metastases and M–1 means that metastases have

been located. The disease is classified under these headings to permit standardization of treatment and comparison between groups.

193   Increase in size, ulceration, deepening colour, itching, bleeding or a halo of pigmentation are all reasons to suspect malignant melanoma in a pre-existing mole.

194   The diagnosis is confirmed histologically and this should be done by excision biopsy with at least a centimetre margin. The surgeon is prepared to proceed to a much wider clearance as soon as the diagnosis is known.

195   Age, sunshine, irradiation and exposure of the skin to chemical irritants such as dyes, tar and soot can all predispose to the development of skin cancer. It can also develop in areas of senile kera-tosis or in an ulcer when it is known as Marjolin's ulcer.

196   The ulcer has rolled edges with a pearly appearance and the centre scabs over and breaks down from time to time. They are nearly always on the face, above the level of the mouth and quite commonly near the eye or nose. Local ero-sion (as a rat might gnaw) is a feature, which is why the name 'rodent ulcer' was given to this le-sion, histologically a basal cell carcinoma.

197   The enlargement can be due to malignant dis-ease either primary or secondary, or to infection which may be regional or generalized. Primary malignant conditions of lymph nodes include Hodgkin's disease and other lymphomas, al-though the axilla is one of the less common sites. Breast carcinoma is the commonest cause of secondary malignancy in the axilla. Infections involving the hand or arm may spread via the lymphatics and present with axillary lympha-denitis — cat scratch fever is in this group. Any of the conditions causing generalized lympha-denitis, such as glandular fever, should be in-cluded in the differential diagnosis although other node groups are usually involved.

198   A pharyngeal pouch can give this history, as can a stone in the submandibular duct. The distinction can be made with a carefully taken history. The

salivary gland swelling is due to salivation alone and it resolves spontaneously whereas a pouch fills with food during a meal and the swelling persists until this is regurgitated or emptied in some way.

199 The differential diagnosis includes primary or secondary malignancy and infection, which is likely to be in the area of the lymphatic drainage. Hodgkin's disease and the lymphomas often present this way. Primary carcinoma of the larynx, nasopharynx, tongue and thryoid are among the causes of secondary malignancy. Any infection in the drainage area can cause this; tuberculosis should not be forgotten.

200 The commonest causes of a tender lump in the groin are strangulated hernia and inflamed lymph nodes. A femoral hernia should always be considered and, of the groin herniae, is the most likely to present in this way. Lymphadenitis or abscess formation may follow infection somewhere in the limb. Less common causes include malignancy, an ectopic testis and femoral artery aneurysm.

201 This was the first human tumour in which there appeared to be a transmissible causative agent. The tumour is only found in areas which share a particular climate and have in common the malaria mosquito which might act as a vector.

202 Torsion of the testis and acute epididymo-orchitis are two conditions that present in this way. The differential diagnosis is usually difficult so the rule is that all tender scrotal swellings should be seen by a surgeon with a view to immediate surgical exploration. However, over the age of about 25 torsion does not occur, so exploration is not necessary in this age group. A less common condition is torsion of the hydatid of Morgagni.

HERNIA

203 The pubic tubercle and the pubic crest medial to it are the surface landmarks of the superficial inguinal ring. The lateral crus is attached to the pubic tubercle which is palpated by invaginating the scrotum behind the cord. The triangular shaped 'ring' lies immediately above and medial

to it with the pubic crest forming its inferior border.

204   The deep ring is bounded laterally and inferiorly by transversus muscle and its attachment to the inguinal ligament. Above and medially is the transversalis fascia. Medially the fascia is condensed over the inferior epigastric vessels which are an important surgical landmark.

205   The spermatic cord includes the vas deferens with its artery and lymphatics, the testicular artery, accompanying sympathetic fibres and the pampiniform plexus of veins. The cord has three coverings: the internal spermatic fascia derived from the transversalis fascia; the cremasteric fascia from the external oblique; and the external spermatic fascia from the external oblique aponeurosis. The cord is not really complete until it leaves the superficial ring.

206   Anteriorly is the inguinal ligament, posteriorly the thickened periosteum of the superior pubic ramus and medially, filling the angle between the two is the pectineal part of the inguinal ligament. Laterally is the femoral vein.

207   A hernia is an abnormal protrusion of an organ or other contents of a body compartment through the wall which normally contains them.

208   A hernia is more likely to strangulate if the neck is small and has unyielding boundaries.

209   Indirect and direct inguinal, and femoral herniae.

210   The direct hernia comes through a diffuse weakness in the abdominal wall — in that sense its route is direct. The indirect hernia traverses the inguinal canal and has an oblique or indirect route.

211   Inguinal herniae are commoner than femoral and represent about 95% in men and 80% in women. Of inguinal herniae the majority are indirect.

212   Inguinal hernia is the commonest inguinoscrotal swelling. This must be differentiated from the 'juvenile' hydrocele which transilluminates and in which there is no cough impulse.

114

213 The indirect hernia passes into the preformed sac which is unobliterated processus vaginalis and therefore can be regarded as basically a congenital abnormality. The direct hernia is through an area of abdominal wall weakness which is acquired.

214 Femoral hernia is bilateral in 20%, indirect inguinal hernia in 30% and direct hernia in 50% of cases.

215 An indirect inguinal hernia.

216 Epigastric hernia occurs between the recti, through the linea alba above the umbilicus. A more diffuse bulge in the midline may be due to divarication of the recti. Umbilical hernia occurs in infants while the adult hernia is usually para-umbilical. Any abdominal incision may be the site of an incisional hernia. Obturator hernia occurs through the obturator foramen and is usually very difficult to detect clinically. Rarer herniae include the Spigelian hernia (which emerges just lateral to the rectus muscle) and the lumbar hernia (which protrudes through a small defect bounded by the iliac crest, the external oblique and the latissimus dorsi muscles).

217 Exomphalos is a congenital abnormality in which the mid-gut fails to return to the coelomic cavity during intra-uterine life and remains at birth as a large hernia.

218 More than 90% disappear before the baby is a year old.

219 An incisional hernia is due to disruption of the deeper layers of a laparotomy wound usually in the early postoperative period. The abdominal contents are retained only by the skin sutures and bulge later as a hernia. Infection or poor tech-nique may be responsible. Modern methods of mass closure or early recognition and resuture of deep dehiscence may prevent herniation later.

220 This term implies the simple transfixation of the neck and excision of the sac as opposed to any form of repair or reinforcement of the associated anatomy which would constitute herniorrhaphy.

221 Inguinal herniae have traditionally been repaired by strengthening the outer layers of the abdominal wall whilst more recent laparoscopic techniques work by strengthening the preperitoneal layers. The traditional repair involves entering the inguinal canal by opening the external oblique, identifying the cord structures and examining them for the presence of an indirect sac. This is opened to examine its contents and then either excised after reducing the contents or, in the case of a sliding hernia, is reduced and the deep ring is tightened. The weak area of Hasselbach's triangle bordered by the inguinal ligament below, the inferior epigastric vessels medially and the conjoint tendon above, is then strengthened by a variety of techniques. The Bassini and Shouldice techniques seek to approximate the inguinal ligament and the external oblique. The Maloney darn technique and the Lichenstein mesh repair introduce loose synthetic material to this area to stimulate the development of a strong fibrous wall. The most popular laparoscopic tehnique is the transabdominal preperitoneal technique (TAPP). From the abdominal cavity, the hernial opening is identified and the peritoneum opened to allow the introduction of a mesh which is stapled in place and the peritoneum is then closed over the top of the mesh.

222 When a viscus is not lying within the sac but has slid down retroperitoneally and forms the posterior wall, this is called a sliding hernia. The viscus involved is typically the caecum on the right and the sigmoid colon on the left. Sometimes the term hernia-en-glissade is used.

223 Umbilical hernia occurs in children whilst para-umbilical hernia occurs in adults. In umbilical hernia the umbilicus is everted and symmetrical, whilst in para-umbilical hernia the sac protrudes beside the umbilicus making it appear asymmetrical.

224 No. The overall recurrence rate in the UK is probably of the order of 10% with most recurrences being evident within a year. Specialist centres achieve recurrence rates of less than 1%. It is hoped that the introduction of new techniques such as the Lichenstein mesh repair will reduce the recurrence rate in the UK.

225 Often with great difficulty! As both may occur below and medial to the pubic tubercle, be very tender and come on relatively quickly, they may sometimes only be distinguished at operation. If the swellings are bilateral, of short duration, associated with perineal sepsis and there are other enlarged groin nodes, the diagnosis is likely to be inguinal lymphadenopathy and should settle with antibiotics. If the swelling is tender and doubt exists about the diagnosis, then exploration is required.

226 Irreducibility means that the hernia cannot be reduced. When this is a long-standing problem and painless, the hernia is referred to as incarcerated. If acutely painful, irreducible herniae require urgent surgery whilst incarcerated ones do not. Strangulation means that the blood supply of the hernia is compromised. Obstruction means that the bowel lumen is occluded within the hernia.

227 The risk of strangulation is highest in femoral hernia and is greater in indirect than direct inguinal hernia. The anatomy of the neck is responsible for these differences.

228 Femoral herniae are particularly liable to strangulate and may go unrecognized even after the onset of complications. Strangulation is particularly likely because of the nature of its neck, while the tendency to go unrecognized is a consequence of its usually small size and its occurrence in fat, old women.

229 Richter's hernia, usually femoral, contains a knuckle of strangulated bowel, but the lumen remains unobstructed as not all the circumference is involved. Littré's hernia contains a Meckel's diverticulum. Maydl's hernia or 'hernia-in-W' contains two loops of bowel and it is the intervening loop hidden inside the abdomen that is strangulated.

230 When the contents do not include the full circumference of a loop of bowel there may be strangulation without obstruction. The ischaemic contents may be omentum or only part of the bowel wall as in Richter's hernia.

231 Patients for day surgery need to be fit and well and to have adequate social backup. Before scheduling a day case procedure, a general enquiry is therefore made about other medical conditions as well as home conditions. Patients must be weighed and their blood pressure taken. Older patients also need an estimation of their blood count and an electrocardiogram.

232 Patients can return to work within a week of their hernia surgery. Traditionally doctors have advised long periods of rest after such surgery, but several studies have shown no increased incidence of recurrence in patients encouraged to return immediately to work. Patients are not so good at applying the brakes in their cars following hernia surgery and should be warned about this; they certainly shouldn't drive home on the day of their operation. They should only drive when they feel fit enough to do so.

ALIMENTARY TRACT (EXCLUDING LARGE BOWEL)

The mouth and salivary glands

233 She has oral candidiasis, otherwise known as thrush. This is a fungal infection, due to *Candida albicans*. It is best treated with nystatin or amphotericin lozenges, continued for at least 48 hours after disappearance of the lesions. This infection is sometimes a sequel to broad spectrum antibiotic therapy and withdrawal of such treatment should be considered if candidiasis develops.

234 At first, besides its presence on self-examination, cancer of the tongue may cause the patient no symptoms. Later pain develops, both locally and perhaps referred to the ear. There may be excessive salivation, bleeding, reduced movement causing dysphagia and dysphonia, marked halitosis and, if lymphatic spread has occurred, a lump in the neck. On examination, the lesion usually has the typical features of a squamous cell carcinoma — a very firm ulcer with a rolled edge; alternative appearances include a warty outgrowth and an ill-defined indurated mass in the tongue.

235 A tongue tie prevents protrusion of the tongue due to a tight fraenum — the thin fold of mucosa and connective tissue connecting the tongue to the floor of the mouth. The condition is often blamed for delays in speech development and difficulties with feeding, but it rarely causes such problems.

236 A mucus retention cyst is caused by obstruction of the small accessory salivary glands in the mucosa inside the lips and mouth. This requires either excision or marsupialization.

237 He has probably developed suppurative parotitis. One or both parotid glands become the site of acute suppurative infection due to dehydration and poor oral hygiene, leading to blockage of the parotid duct with debris and infection in the obstructed gland. It was much more common when postoperative care, in particular fluid replacement, was less satisfactory than it is today.

238 The facial, lingual and hypoglossal nerves. During parotid surgery, the facial nerve can be damaged as it runs through the substance of the gland, in which it divides into its five branches. Division of the trunk or branches produces corresponding paralysis of one side of the face. During exposure of the submandibular gland, the mandibular branch of the facial nerve can be damaged causing ugly droop of the corner of the mouth. The lingual and hypoglossal nerves can be damaged during mobilization of this gland, causing unilateral anaesthesia and paralysis of the tongue respectively.

239 The parotid duct opens beneath a small papilla on the inside of the cheek opposite the second upper molar tooth, while the submandibular duct opens on the summit of the sublingual papilla, a few millimetres lateral to the fraenum of the tongue.

240 The parotid gland is invested in an unyielding capsule, derived from the deep cervical fascia. The capsule is incapable of much expansion, so that great pressure builds up within it as the gland swells due to acute inflammation, causing severe pain.

241 The commonest parotid tumour is variously known as a mixed parotid tumour, myoepithelioma or pleomorphic adenoma. The first of these names was the original and was coined because this tumour was thought to be of mixed cell origin as it appeared to contain epithelial and cartilaginous elements. The 'cartilage' has since been shown to be mucin, probably secreted by myoepithelial cells around the acini, hence the second name. The third name, pleomorphic adenoma, describes adequately the microscopic appearances and is the one in most common usage. This tumour is usually benign and is best treated by superficial parotidectomy, preserving the facial nerve. This procedure is preferred to enucleation of the tumour as the latter is likely to leave islands of growth and is also more likely to lead to operative damage to the facial nerve.

242 After superficial parotidectomy, the recurrence rate is about 5%. However, after removal of recurrent tumours, they recur again in 25% of cases. 2 to 3% of pleomorphic adenomas become malignant and recurrence after removal of these tumours is about 35% and double this after treatment of recurrence.

243 The medical conditions which cause salivary gland enlargement are mumps, suppurative parotitis, Sjögren's syndrome, Mikulicz disease, sarcoidosis and sialectasis.

244 This is not fully understood. They are usually composed of calcium and magnesium phosphates, like the tartar that forms on teeth. This may form around minute food particles or shed cells which find their way into the duct.

245 The stone is removed under local or general anaesthesia. The stone is immobilized by a suture and the duct opened at the site of the stone, allowing it to escape. Some stones may necessitate gland excision.

The oesophagus

246 The most important factor is the presence of a short segment of intra-abdominal oesophagus

which is kept closed by positive intra-abdominal pressure. Other factors are the 'flap-valve' effect of the oesophagogastric angle; the high pressure zone in the lower oesophagus, in which there appears to be a physiologically active sphincter mechanism; the rosette-like folds of gastric mucosa plugging the cardia; and the right crus of the diaphragm encircling the oesophageal hiatus.

247 The oesophagus is lined throughout by stratified, non-keratinizing squamous epithelium. Deep to this is a wide submucosal layer, containing mucous glands; the muscle layer is made up of circular and longitudinal layers which are striated in the upper third, smooth in the lower third and mixed in the middle. Between the muscle layers is the myenteric nerve plexus.

248 Dysphagia means difficulty in swallowing. The most important and common causes are carcinoma of the oesophagus, benign peptic stricture due to hiatal hernia and achalasia of the cardia. Other causes include mediastinal malignancy, such as secondary lung cancer, retrosternal goitre, a large pharyngeal pouch, scleroderma and neurological conditions such as bulbar palsy and myasthenia gravis.

249 The first thing to do is to confirm that the patient has carcinoma of the oesophagus by taking a biopsy at endoscopy. The disease then needs staging by ultrasound of the liver, chest X-ray and computerized tomographic (CT) scanning. The patient's general fitness for anaesthesia needs assessment clinically and by measuring their lung function.

250 Potassium tablets in prolonged contact with mucosa anywhere in the alimentary tract will cause ulceration and fibrosis due to the effect of a high local concentration of potassium. Patients with cardiac disease are at particular risk, as enlargement of the left atrium causes pressure on the mid-oesophagus, so that tablets containing potassium may be held up at this level, perhaps producing an oesophageal stricture.

251 This is a squamous cell lesion, more common in men than women and with a peak age incidence between 65 and 75 years. It causes 2500 deaths in

the UK each year. 80% of growths occur in the lower half of the oesophagus. This tumour spreads locally via the submucosal layer, so that the mucosal and external appearance of the oesophagus may give a false impression of the extent of the disease. Lymphatic spread occurs early to nodes in the neck, lung hilum or coeliac group, depending on the site of the primary. Distant, blood-borne spread is not a major feature as patients frequently die before this can occur.

252 The oesophagus can be mobilized in the chest via an abdominal incision or by a minimally invasive technique, then pulled up into the neck to perform an anastomosis without opening the chest. Radical radiotherapy, chemotherapy, endoscopic intubation, or laser treatment are alternatives in appropriate circumstances.

253 This is a particularly nasty disease, as the poor prognosis illustrates — only 50–60% are suitable for radical surgery and in these the 2-year survival is only around 25%.

254 Heartburn is a pain radiating up behind the sternum into the neck caused by acid reflux from stomach into oesophagus. Having reassured the patient that they are not having a heart attack you should advise them to lose weight, eat small, regular meals, to prop the head of the bed up and not to smoke or drink. Drug treatment is by acid reduction with gaviscon (a mixture of alginates and antacids), omeprazole or high dose ranitidine and motility agents to encourage gastric emptying such as cisapride. Surgery by Nissen fundoplication is reserved for those cases with complications such as bleeding or stenosis, or failure to resolve symptoms by medical treatments.

255 The commonest type is the sliding hernia in which the cardia moves up into the chest, with a variable portion of the stomach. The less common varieties are the para-oesophageal or rolling hernia, in which the fundus of the stomach enters the chest while the cardia remains in place, and the mixed type, a combination of the sliding and rolling varieties. Most hiatal herniae are asymptomatic. Sliding hernia may present with symptoms due to gastro-oesophageal reflux, that is, heartburn and flatulence. Rolling hernia does not

cause reflux but may produce anaemia due to gastric ulcer in the herniated stomach, while sometimes the latter becomes obstructed or strangulated, indicated by chest or upper abdominal pain and shock.

256   Such patients may develop peptic oesophagitis due to acid reflux, and in a proportion of patients going on to produce ulceration, fibrosis and stricture, always at the junction of gastric and oesophageal mucosa. Refluxed material can spill over into the larynx, sometimes leading to aspiration pneumonia. Finally, some believe that carcinoma can arise at the cardia in patients with hiatal hernia.

257   Surgery is indicated for the complications of reflux oesophagitis such as severe haemorrhage, peptic stricture and for failed medical treatment. Surgery can be performed via the abdomen or less commonly via the chest. The most popular technique is the Nissen fundoplication which may be performed laparoscopically ('a lap wrap'). This involves wrapping the fundus of the stomach around the oesophagus, combined with narrowing of the oesophageal hiatus. Other techniques include the introduction of an Angelchick prosthesis around the intra-abdominal oesophagus. The transthoracic Belsey repair is used less frequently these days.

258   Achalasia is a condition in which the cardia fails to relax as a bolus of food approaches and is due to absence or paucity of ganglion cells in the myenteric plexus. The condition usually presents at the age of 20 to 40, and the typical symptoms are painless dysphagia for both solids and liquids and a sensation of food sticking behind the lower sternum. The patient has to eat slowly, perhaps using Valsalva's manoeuvre to empty the oesophagus forcibly into the stomach. There is often a history of frequent regurgitation, sometimes with choking and evidence of aspiration pneumonia. Barium swallow shows a greatly dilated, cucumber-shaped oesophagus, with no normal movements. Treatment is surgical — Heller's operation is performed in which the muscle, but not the mucosa, of the distal oesophagus is incised longitudinally through either an abdominal or a thoracic approach.

259 The site depends on the aetiology. The common-
     est benign stricture is due to an acid/peptic reflux
     in hiatal hernia and occurs at the junction of
     oesophageal and gastric mucosa, that is, usually
     in the distal third. Strictures due to ingestion of
     strong acid or alkali are often multiple, while
     'postassium stricture' in cardiac patients is in the
     mid zone where the enlarged left atrium presses
     on the oesophagus. Treatment of peptic stricture
     is normally conservative initially, with cimetidine
     and dilatation of the stricture endoscopically. If
     this is unsuccessful, surgery for the hiatal hernia
     and occasionally, resection of the stricture, are re-
     quired.

260 This emergency is usually first dealt with by the
     insertion of a Sengstaken-Blakemore tube, which
     applies local pressure to the oesophageal varices
     and their feeding veins in the gastric fundus.
     An alternative initial procedure is the intravenous
     injection of Pitressin. After initial control,
     endoscopic injection sclerotherapy is effective in
     preventing early rebleeding. More invasive mea-
     sures include trans-abdominal devascularization
     of the gastric fundus, with staple-gun division and
     anastomosis of the lower oesophagus; trans-
     thoracic underrunning of the varices; and porta-
     systemic shunting.

The stomach

261 Any of the structures related to the stomach can
     become involved with gastric cancer by direct
     spread. Anteriorly or above, the liver, biliary tree,
     abdominal wall, oesophagus and diaphragm may
     be invaded, while behind lie the pancreas, trans-
     verse mesocolon, spleen and posterior abdominal
     wall. Inferior spread can affect the transverse co-
     lon. Direct spread into several of these organs
     produces characteristic features. For instance,
     oesophageal involvement causes dysphagia, while
     invasion of the transverse colon may produce a
     gastrocolic fistula and hence the vomiting of fae-
     ces. Posterior spread into the pancreas or poste-
     rior wall musculature can produce severe back
     pain, so that this is a sinister symptom in a case of
     suspected gastric cancer.

262 The stomach has a copious arterial supply via four main arteries, the left and right gastrics, and the left and right gastro-epiploics. The left gastric artery is the largest of these; it arises directly from the coeliac axis, and passes to the upper lesser curve where it divides into superior and inferior branches. The right gastric artery usually arises from the common hepatic artery or one of its major branches and reaches the lower lesser curve near the upper border of the pylorus. The left gastro-epiploic artery arises from the splenic artery in the splenic hilum, and runs down the greater curve of the stomach to anastomose with the right gastro-epiploic artery which arises from the gastroduodenal artery near the inferior border of the pylorus. Besides these four major vessels, several short gastric arteries arise from the splenic artery at the splenic hilum to supply the upper greater curve. All these vessels give many anterior and posterior branches which anastomose profusely within the wall of the stomach. Veins corresponding to each of these arteries drain into the portal system.

263 The stomach has two main functions — acid/peptic digestion of food and temporary storage of partly digested food prior to its discharge into the duodenum for further digestion. In addition it produces intrinsic factor which binds vitamin B_{12} ready for absorption in the distal ileum.

264 Gastrin is produced by the G-cells in the gastric antrum. Hydrochloric acid is secreted by the parietal cells in the mucosa of the body of the stomach. Pepsin is not produced as such by the gastric mucosa — pepsinogen is secreted by the zymogen cells of the body of the stomach and converted to pepsin by the action of acid in the gastric lumen.

265 Gastric acid secretion is induced by the thought and taste of food which cause vagal stimulation of the stomach; and by the entry of food into the stomach, causing gastrin release from the antrum; and by the entry of food and its digestive products into the small bowel, acting by release of intestinal gastrin. This stimulates the proton pump which secretes hydrogen ions in the gastric mucosa of the body of the stomach.

266 Gastric acid secretion can be reduced by drugs; very occasionally surgical reduction will be used, mainly in the treatment of complications of peptic ulcer disease. Cimetidine and ranitidine, both H_2 receptor antagonists, act by blocking histamine induction of acid release, the final common pathway for all modes of gastric acid secretion. Omeprazole and lansoprazole act directly to inhibit the proton pump. These approaches have been a major step forward in the medical treatment of peptic ulcer disease. Surgical methods of reducing gastric acid secretion are vagotomy in its various forms; antrectomy which removes the gastrin-producing area of the stomach; and total gastrectomy, which removes the acid-producing area as well as the antrum and is the only procedure which can totally abolish acid production.

267 Gastric cancer usually develops insidiously, so that it is usually advanced by the time of diagnosis. Most patients give a story of persistent indigestion with anorexia and weight loss. The patient is often anaemic and may have an epigastric mass. Sometimes the lesion will cause dysphagia at an early stage, due to involvement of the cardio-oesophageal junction, while in a minority haematemesis or perforation will be the mode of presentation. In a few, spread beyond the stomach will lead to ascites due to peritoneal spread; jaundice due to liver secondaries; or a lump in the neck due to lymphatic spread (Troisier's sign).

268 Gastric cancer arises more frequently in patients with pernicious anaemia. It is apparent that gastric cancer may arise from areas of intestinal metaplasia within the stomach and that, in the rare instance when true adenomas are present in the stomach, these may become malignant.

269 'Hour glass' stomach is a deformity of the stomach related to long-standing benign ulceration producing a narrowing in the centre of the stomach leaving two pouches on either side resembling an hour glass. 'Leather bottle' stomach or linitis plastica is a form of carcinoma of the stomach in which the malignant infiltration makes the stomach rigid, contracted and undistensible.

270 Operations for gastric cancer may be radical or palliative. Radical operations, performed in the hope of cure, involve removal of all or most of the stomach, together with its lymphatic drainage and any locally involved adjacent tissue, followed by a reconstruction to restore continuity. Palliative surgery may amount to removal of the primary — as a subtotal gastrectomy — in cases where distant spread has rendered the patient incurable; sometimes the tumour is irremovably invading locally, so that a gastrojejunostomy bypassing the growth is all that is possible. Radical surgery is feasible in about 50% of cases and palliative surgery in about 20%, while in the remainder the growth is beyond any surgical help at the time of laparotomy.

271 In general no — the median survival of all cases is less than 6 months. About 10% of all patients survive for 5 years and even if radical resection has been possible, the corresponding figure is only about 30%. The only group of patients with a good prognosis are those with the lesion called 'early gastric cancer' in which the tumour is confined to the mucosa and submucosa, with or without lymphatic involvement — in this group, the 5-year survival is at least 70% after radical surgery.

272 Weight loss in gastric ulcer patients is common due to the tendency for them to avoid eating for fear of bringing on their pain. However, the possibility must be borne in mind that the ulcer might be a malignancy and that this may be the cause of the weight loss.

273 Back pain in such a patient suggests penetration of the ulcer through the posterior wall of the stomach, into structures in the stomach bed, usually the pancreas. Penetration can occur with benign or malignant ulcers, so back pain does not necessarily indicate carcinoma.

274 Unlike duodenal ulcer, gastric ulcers are sometimes malignant — clinical and radiological evidence alone cannot exclude carcinoma. Therefore, before beginning a trial of medical treatment for any gastric ulcer, endoscopy should be carried

out to allow careful, direct inspection of the lesion and, more importantly, multiple biopsy of the edge and base of the ulcer.

275 Assuming that the ulcer has been carefully investigated by X-ray, endoscopy and multiple biopsy, it is safe to try to heal it by medical means. The patient should first be told to stop smoking and to take a regular diet. Medication may take various forms — in particular cimetidine may be prescribed to decrease acid secretion and carbenoxolone or bismuth compounds may be used to aid the protection of the mucosa, either by an effect on the gastric mucus or directly. If the ulcer has not healed within 8 to 12 weeks, or if complications supervene, operation should be advised.

276 There are three, possibly four complications of gastric ulcer; haemorrhage, perforation, stenosis of the stomach at the level of the ulcer and malignant change. The last of these is questionable as a complication of benign ulcer — some would say that 'ulcer cancers' are malignant from the outset.

277 The features of a gastric ulcer that should be checked when deciding whether it might be malignant are its site and its profile. While ulcers sited on the lesser curve can be benign or malignant, ulcers elsewhere in the stomach should be viewed with particular suspicion. If the ulcer is shown in profile, one should check whether the base lies outside the contour of the stomach, or within it suggesting ulceration of a cancer encroaching on the lumen. However, neither of these signs is sufficiently specific, so that endoscopy and biopsy remain necessary.

278 This is a condition in which multiple shallow ulcers, usually less than 5 mm in diameter, develop in the stomach. There may be a few, or the whole mucosa may be affected. The intervening mucosa is often oedematous and engorged, and there may be areas of submucosal haemorrhage. This condition usually develops in patients very ill from some other problem, and is often encountered in the Intensive Care Unit. Patients with severe burns, head injuries, strokes, overwhelming sepsis, respiratory, renal or liver

failure are all prone to erosive gastritis. It can also occur in alcohol abuse or after the use of aspirin and other anti-inflammatory drugs.

279　The major element of the management of a case of bleeding erosive gastritis is circulatory support — the bleeding is usually not severe and can be expected to stop spontaneously in most cases. Blood loss is replaced; cimetidine is usually given intravenously, though there is little evidence of its positive value in this situation. If bleeding continues, vasopressin may be given, while therapeutic embolization may be considered if this fails. Surgery is the last resort, as it is often ineffective in this condition and carries a high mortality; if surgery is necessary, vagotomy with partial gastrectomy is probably the procedure of choice.

280　The commonest causes of upper gastro-intestinal haemorrhage are duodenal ulcer, gastric ulcer and actue gastric erosions — these lesions account for more than 80% of cases. Mallory-Weiss mucosal tears at the cardia, oesophageal varices and gastric neoplasms account for most of the remainder.

281　Early endoscopy is popular among clinicians treating upper gastro-intestinal haemorrhage because it provides a definitive diagnosis in most cases, allowing treatment to be more precisely tailored to the underlying cause. In particular, it picks out those patients in whom bleeding is unlikely to respond to resuscitation alone (oesophageal varices) and vice versa (gastric erosions). However, as yet there is no convincing evidence that this apparently useful tool sufficiently improves management to reduce overall mortality in upper GI bleeding.

282　Most bleeding peptic ulcers will stop bleeding without any specific treatment. Such patients are admitted to hospital, given a blood transfusion and endoscoped to confirm the diagnosis. If the ulcer is seen to be at risk of rebleeding at endoscopy, it can be injected with adrenalin. If the patient does rebleed they may require surgery which involves underrunning the ulcer with a stitch or in some cases gastrectomy.

283 Most anaemia following gastrectomy is related to iron deficiency. This is thought to be due to reduced iron absorption rather than to the development of a stomal ulcer. Vitamin B_{12} deficiency is inevitable after total gastrectomy and so is usually prevented by injections of the vitamin every 3 months.

The duodenum

284 By convention, the term 'penetration' implies the extension of peptic ulceration through the posterior wall, as opposed to anterior perforation into the peritoneal cavity. Therefore the structures lying behind the first part of the duodenum may be penetrated — these are the gastroduodenal artery and its branches, which may bleed and the pancreas which may cause back pain.

285 Duodenal diverticulum causes no symptoms and is therefore of very little significance itself, but because it usually lies immediately next to the distal end of the common bile duct, it can make ERCP difficult.

286 The duodenal mucosa secretes cholecystokinin-pancreozymin, secretin and enterogastrone. All three are released into the portal vein when the initial products of digestion leave the stomach. CCK-PZ stimulates the gall-bladder to contract and the pancreas to secrete enzymes into the pancreatic juice; secretin stimulates the pancreas to release water and electrolytes into the duct system; while enterogastrone inhibits gastric secretion and motility, probably by inhibiting gastrin release.

287 There are two protective mechanisms — the mucus barrier and neutralization of acid by the alkaline bile and pancreatic juice; secretion of both is stimulated by the passage of acid gastric content into the duodenum.

288 Duodenal ulcers may be caused by *Helicobacter pylorii* weakening the mucosal barrier against gastric acid. Its presence may be demonstrated in biopsies from the gastric antrum by culturing it, identifying it on histological biopsies and by the urease breath test.

289 The usual symptoms of duodenal ulcer are epigastric pain which comes on several hours after meals, that is, prior to the next meal, which is relieved by food or alkalis and which may also wake the patient in the early hours, when again it is relieved by nourishment. These symptoms are usually periodic, troubling the patient for a month or two, followed by a remission of similar length. The patient is more often male than female, aged 25 to 50, probably smokes, and is likely to have a stressful existence, either because of his personality or his job.

290 Duodenal ulcers in the anterior wall of the duodenum erode through into the peritoneal cavity and so cause peritonitis. Those in the posterior wall erode backwards into the gastroduodenal artery and so cause haemorrhage.

291 The first line treatment in the patient with a simple duodenal ulcer is usually a 4-week course of an H_2 antagonist such as ranitidine or a proton pump inhibitor such as omeprazole. This is in addition to the usual advice about diet, stopping smoking and reducing alcohol intake. Whilst usually curative, the longer term relapse rate is high due to underlying infection by *Helicobacter pylorii*. This bacteria may be treated blindly at first presentation, following relapse, or after confirmation by endoscopy and biopsy or by breath testing.

292 *Helicobacter pylorii* can be treated by 'triple therapy' with Denol (tri-potassium di-citrate bismuthate) together with metronidazole and another antibiotic such as amoxycillin. These three drugs are given for between 2 and 4 weeks. However, compliance is a problem with such a regimen and some doctors prefer to treat it with omeprazole and amoxycillin, or clarithromycin. Treatment is usually given for patients with duodenal ulcer in whom *Helicobacter pylorii* has been identified in endoscopic samples or by breath testing, but treatment can be given blindly to all patients presenting with a duodenal ulcer.

293 Surgery is indicated in duodenal ulcer if medical management fails to produce adequate symptomatic relief, or if any of the complications arise (perforation, major haemorrhage or pyloric stenosis).

294 Nowadays most surgeons perform some form of vagotomy for duodenal ulcer — this may be a truncal or selective vagotomy with either a pyloroplasty or gastro-enterostomy or a highly selective vagotomy without a drainage procedure. In some circumstances, particularly when a duodenal ulcer is bleeding, a partial gastrectomy may be appropriate. Some surgeons combine the two types of operation by performing vagotomy and antrectomy, which has the lowest rate of ulcer recurrence.

295 A pyloroplasty is an operation in which the lumen of the pylorus is enlarged. For example the pylorus may be divided longitudinally and then sutured transversely. It allows drainage of the duodenum after the vagus nerve is divided in a truncal vagotomy. Alternatives are a gastro-jejunostomy or a highly selective vagotomy in which the nerves to the pylorus are preserved, so that a drainage procedure is not needed.

296 The main long-term complications are recurrent ulcer and diarrhoea, both more common after vagotomy than gastrectomy; dumping, anaemia, bilious vomiting and gastric cancer are more common after gastrectomy than vagotomy.

The pancreas

297 The pancreas has an autonomic nerve supply, both sympathetic and parasympathetic, arising from the coeliac plexus, around the origin of the coeliac artery. This assumes clinical importance in patients with pancreatic cancer, in whom percutaneous destruction of the coeliac plexus using injections of alcohol or phenol may be used for pain relief.

298 The major factors in the promotion of pancreatic exocrine secretion are the hormones secretin and cholecystokinin-pancreozymin. They are released into the portal blood by duodenal and upper small bowel mucosa when acid and initial products of digestion leave the stomach. Secretin promotes water and electrolyte secretion, while CCK-PZ promotes enzyme release into pancreatic juice. As gastric emptying ceases, hormone

drive on the pancreas diminishes, so that secretion is inhibited.

299 Tumours of the pancreas are usually primary tumours and mostly malignant. The commonest is an adenocarcinoma of the head of the pancreas. The endocrine cells can give rise to tumours which are usually benign such as a vipoma, gastrinoma, glucagonoma and insulinoma.

300 While the classical triad of weight loss, jaundice and pain can occur in any case of pancreatic cancer, jaundice is more frequent when the growth is in the head and pain is more common in body or tail lesions. Lesions in the head often involve the bile duct, so jaundice is present on first visit in 80%; in more distal lesions, jaundice does not develop until there are liver metastases. Pain is less common at initial presentation in head lesions because jaundice develops early, leading to earlier presentation compared to body and tail growths, which have frequently spread into the posterior abdominal wall when first seen.

301 Sometimes. As with any tumour, proof depends on acquiring tissue diagnosis. In pancreatic cancer, cytological specimens may be recovered by endoscopic brushing or collection of pancreatic juice, or by ultrasound-directed percutaneous needle aspiration of the lesion. Other diagnostic methods, including various radiological approaches, can only provide suggestive evidence.

302 Whipple's operation, otherwise known as pancreaticoduodenectomy, is an operation to remove the head of the pancreas and the duodenum and it is performed for potentially curable tumours of this region. The high recurrence rate and operative mortality when this is performed for carcinoma of the head of pancreas, have caused this operation to fall into disfavour, except for carcinoma of the ampulla of the bile duct.

303 This term should be used only in patients with pancreatic pain and with evidence of pancreatic exocrine insufficiency in whom the pancreas has been shown radiologically or at operation to be the site of disease. It may be complicated by recurrent episodes of acute pancreatitis. The

pathological process is progressive, irreversible inflammation, usually caused by alcohol or by gall-stone disease. Initially there is plugging of minor ducts causing dilatation and fibrosis, the process later spreading to the major ducts.

304 Patients suffering from chronic pancreatitis require a high protein, high calorie diet, and must stop drinking. Further treatment depends on symptoms — malabsorption can be treated with pancreatic enzyme replacement tablets, and diabetes is managed appropriately. If pain or jaundice are the main problems, surgery must be considered. ERCP should be performed to determine the anatomy of the diseased pancreas and the state of the bile duct. Surgery aims at decompressing the obstructed pancreatic duct, usually by distal resection and drainage into the small bowel, or by longitudinal pancreatojejunostomy.

305 This is a collection of pancreatic secretion and inflammatory exudate in the lesser sac in some cases of acute or chronic pancreatitis, which may be responsible for continued discomfort and debility; it is lined by fibrous and inflammatory tissue rather than epithelium — hence the term 'pseudocyst'. Its presence may be suspected from the history and a mass in the epigastrium, while confirmation is usually obtained by ultrasound examination. Some pseudocysts resolve spontaneously but the larger, symptomatic ones require surgery. The cyst is approached through the stomach, a wide opening being made into the cyst through the posterior wall — cystogastrostomy. The cyst contents drain into the stomach, after which the opening in the stomach closes spontaneously.

The liver

306 The liver is made up of eight segments based on the divisions of the hepatic artery and the portal vein. Segments 5–8 make up the right half of the liver and segments 1–4 the left half (a rather larger structure than the left lobe of the liver). Their clinical relevance is that resection of a segment of the liver is possible in the same way as resecting lobes of the lung.

307 During the usual lateral approach, the lung may be punctured if the patient has not breathed out fully. The gall-bladder, the structures in the free edge of the lesser omentum, the duodenum and the hepatic flexure of the colon can all be damaged if the needle is pushed in too far and especially if an anterior approach is used. The kidney may also be injured.

308 Liver secondaries can be suspected clinically if the liver is enlarged and irregular; they can be seen at operation; they can be detected by ultrasound, isotope scanning or CT scan; but they can be proven only on histological examination of material taken by needle biopsy or at operation. Changes in blood tests, particularly the serum alkaline phosphatase and bilirubin, occur only when there is massive replacement of liver tissue by secondary deposits and are thus a late indicator.

309 It is sometimes possible to remove solitary secondaries curatively, while multiple, symptomatic deposits are sometimes amenable to palliative treatment. Curative resection should only be attempted for colorectal secondaries and then only if investigations suggest that the disease is localized to one lobe, in which case a wedge or even a lobe can be resected. There is no prospect of cure with other primary sites. Palliation of pain due to secondaries from any site can sometimes be achieved by the radiologist using embolization via an arterial catheter. Chemotherapy using 5-fluorouracil and folinic acid may delay and/or palliate the symptoms of colorectal metastases which are not surgically removable.

310 The most common predisposing factor is cirrhosis, especially when induced by alcohol or hepatitis B. Very important factors elsewhere in the world are aflatoxin contamination of food in Southern Africa and liver fluke infestation in the Far East.

311 Hydatid disease — infestation with *Echinococcus granulosus*. This organism is ingested by humans via the faecal–oral route from dogs which excrete the eggs, having eaten offal from sheep already infested with *Echinococcus*. The organisms travel

via the portal system to the liver, where they form cysts, inside which small daughter cysts proliferate. Other organs, particularly the lung, can become infested.

312 Liver abscesses in Britain are almost always pyogenic, and occur most frequently in patients with biliary disease or some form of pre-existing malignancy or an inflammatory condition such as diverticular disease.

313 The two essentials in the treatment of unilocular liver abscesses are drainage and adequate antibiotics. Drainage may be by closed aspiration via a tube inserted with ultrasound or CT guidance, or by open operation. Antibiotics should initially be a wide spectrum combination, such as tobramycin, ampicillin and metronidazole, until examination of the pus allows a more specific approach.

314 The surgeon most commonly becomes involved in the management of cirrhosis when the patient develops a gastro-intestinal haemorrhage. After diagnosing oesophageal varices, initial treatment is by tamponade with a Sengstaken tube. Injection sclerotherapy is next used, but if this fails transection of the oesophagus with a stapling instrument may be necessary. Portal systemic shunts have become less popular because of the operative mortality and the high incidence of hepatic encephalopathy. Cirrhosis in patients who are not alcoholics may be an indication for transplantation.

315 Liver transplantation is considered for patients with primary biliary cirrhosis, sclerosing cholangitis, metabolic disorders, posthepatic cirrhosis, drug-induced liver damage, congenital disorders and for primary hepatocellular carcinoma. After permission is given for the donation and death has been confirmed by brain stem tests, the donor is maintained on a ventilator with adequate hydration and dopamine. The donor liver is perfused with an ice-cold preserving solution and maintained cold for up to 16 hours. During removal of the old liver from the recipient, the inferior vena cava and portal vein are occluded impeding venous return. A venous bypass is

therefore established between the upper and lower limbs. The inferior vena cava from the new liver is anastomosed to the inferior vena cava of the recipient, followed by the portal veins. The arterial and biliary anastomoses are next preformed. Immunosuppression is maintained postoperatively with cyclosporin A.

The biliary tree

316   The structures in greatest danger are the extrahepatic biliary tree and the blood vessels supplying the liver. Damage may occur if an adequate view of the various structures is not ensured during dissection — this may be hampered by the build of the patient, poor lighting and inadequate assistance. If unexpected bleeding occurs, blind attempts to stop it can lead to accidental duct injuries. Less commonly, anatomical anomalies lead to mistaken ligation and division of vital ducts or vessels.

317   The distal common bile duct passes behind the pancreas to enter the duodenum, usually in its second part, at the papilla of Vater. As the duct passes through the duodenal wall it is surrounded by a cuff of muscle of variable length, the sphincter of Oddi. In about 75% of individuals the pancreatic duct enters the distal common duct through the sphincter of Oddi; in the remainder it either enters the duct above the sphincter or enters the duodenum separately.

318   Bile is unique in being both an exocrine secretion, playing a role in digestion and a major excretory pathway. The digestive function is played by bile acids and phospholipids, which form micelles or 'packets' of water-insoluble dietary lipids, ready for absorption; in addition bile acids activate pancreatic lipase. Bile contains excreted bilirubin and cholesterol, the latter held in solution by micelle formation with the bile acids and phospholipids.

319   Asymptomatic gall-stones, polyps in the gallbladder wall, cysts of the liver and choledochal cysts may all be found incidentally on an ultrasound scan of the biliary tree. Asymptomatic gallstones and gall-bladder polyps as well as small

simple liver cysts can all be left safely alone. Cysts from hydatid disease and choledochal cysts require surgical treatment.

320 It appears that most gall-stones develop due to changes in the relative proportions of bile acids, phospholipids and cholesterol in the bile. As the latter, which is water-insoluble, is held in solution by aggregation with the other two constituents, increase in cholesterol content or decrease in bile acid content lead to cholesterol microcrystal formation and later to gall-stones. Increased cholesterol content occurs in people on the contraceptive pill or on clofibrate and may also be related to a highly refined Western diet. Bile acid concentration may fall in patients with abnormal enterohepatic circulation, such as those with Crohn's disease or a small bowel fistula. Pigment stones are common in patients with chronic haemolytic disease (in whom bile pigment excretion is excessive) such as sickle-cell anaemia.

321 Gall-stones are commonest in middle-aged, overweight mothers. Typically, the patient complains of postprandial discomfort sometimes amounting to pain, in the epigastrium or right upper quadrant which may radiate to the right scapular area. Symptoms may be especially bad after fatty or fried foods. If gall-stones are confirmed in these people, they are said to be suffering from chronic cholecystitis.

322 Gall-stones most commonly cause biliary colic or acute cholecystitis if they obstruct the drainage of bile from the gall-bladder. If they then pass through the cystic duct into the common bile duct they can cause ascending cholangitis, obstructive jaundice and may cause pancreatitis. Rarer complications include mucocele of the gallbladder, empyema of the gall-bladder, gangrene of the gall-bladder with biliary peritonitis and gall-stone ileus.

323 The diagnosis is confirmed by oral cholecystography or ultrasound. In an oral cholecystogram plain films are taken one day, the patient takes tablets containing an iodine compound that night and further films are taken the next day as the contrast is concentrated in the gall-bladder, if

138

it is functioning. A simpler technique is biliary ultrasonography. This not only allows confirmation of stones in the gall-bladder but also provides information about the bile duct and pancreas and can be used in jaundiced patients. This technique is more liable to error in interpretation of results and hence sometimes less reliable. Another technique sometimes used in acutely ill or jaundiced patients is HIDA-scanning, an intravenous isotope technique in which a radiolabelled substance is rapidly excreted into the bile allowing biliary imaging — 'absence' of a gall-bladder arising from the bile duct suggests cystic duct obstruction.

324 Courvoisier's Law states that, if in a patient with obstructive jaundice the gall-bladder is palpable, then the jaundice is unlikely to be due to gall-stones. The rule is not completely reliable, but it is helpful in distinguishing those patients likely to have malignant causes for their obstructive jaundice, from those in whom the cause is gall-stones.

325 Most gall-bladders are removed laparoscopically although some still require open laparotomy. Patients with symptomatic gall-stones in the absence of acute complications are mostly considered suitable for laparoscopic surgery. Although it will depend on the experience of the operator, if surgery is required in acute cholecystitis, pancreatitis, or the presence of jaundice, morbid obesity, stones in the common bile duct and dense adhesions from previous surgery, then the procedure may be more safely performed 'open'.

326 This is a radiological technique which allows confirmation of the anatomy of the biliary tree prior to division of the presumed cystic duct and demonstrates abnormalities of the extrahepatic duct such as dilatation and duct stones. It is performed by injecting contrast via a small cannula in the cystic duct and exposing three X-ray films after repeated injections, the films being placed in a tunnel under the patient. Operative cholangiography provides a more reliable basis for the decision to explore the bile duct than is possible using clinical data and duct palpation alone, leading to fewer unproductive explorations and lower morbidity.

327 In some patients gall-stones can be removed by
dissolution. Stones consisting mainly of cholesterol can be made to dissolve by giving the bile
acid, chenodeoxycholic acid, orally for long periods. However, this treatment has drawbacks —
the gall-bladder must be functioning; the stones
must not contain calcium, as judged on X-ray and
they should be small; the patient should not be a
young woman likely to become pregnant and
should not have liver disease or be suffering frequent bouts of biliary pain. Furthermore, the
stones are very likely to recur if therapy is
stopped.

328 This term implies jaundice due to mechanical obstruction of the extrahepatic biliary tree. The
commonest causes of obstructive jaundice are
gall-stones in the bile duct, and carcinoma of the
head of pancreas. Less common are carcinoma of
the ampulla of Vater or of the bile duct; traumatic
duct stricture, due to previous surgery; sclerosing
cholangitis; pancreatitis; and parasitic infestation
of the duct. It is very important to differentiate
jaundice due to one of these 'surgical' conditions
from 'cholestatic' jaundice (which is caused by
intrahepatic small duct obstruction due to a drug
reaction, hepatitis or cirrhosis and which has
many of the clinical and biochemical features of
obstruction), as surgery in this group would be
totally inappropriate.

329 This is probably due to the deposition of bile
acids in the skin. Besides the use of conventional
antipruritic treatment, cholestyramine can be
administered which may help by increasing faecal
loss of bile acids.

330 The typical changes in liver function tests in obstructive jaundice (besides a raised bilirubin) are
a markedly raised alkaline phosphatase, with
lesser rises in the hepatocellular enzymes. However, a biochemically 'obstructive' picture is also
found in patients with intrahepatic cholestasis
due to medical causes, so chemistry alone is not
sufficient to prove extrahepatic obstruction.

331 ERCP (endoscopic retrograde cholangiopan-
creatography) can be used both to confirm the
diagnosis and to remove the gall-stones after performing a sphincterotomy at the lower end of the

common bile duct through the endoscope. This is the treatment of choice in older patients unless urgent surgery is indicated for other reasons. In younger patients and when ERCP fails, then an open operation removing the gall-bladder and exploring the common bile duct is performed. A few surgeons now explore the common bile duct through the laparoscope, but at present this is a relatively experimental technique. For very large stones the lithotripter, in conjunction with a sphincterotomy performed at ERCP, may be used. Occasionally biliary bypass may be required by choledochoduodenostomy.

332 This term refers to the renal failure which may develop in the patient undergoing surgery for obstructive jaundice. The exact cause for this problem is not clear, but it seems that the renal tubules are especially sensitive to ischaemic damage in hyperbilirubinaemia and in the endotoxaemia resulting from the poor reticulo-endothelial function of the compromised liver. Prophylaxis involves maintaining diuresis throughout the perioperative period using a fluid load and mannitol infusion; in addition, full antibiotic cover may decrease endotoxaemia.

333 A T-tube is a drainage device used following exploration of the common bile duct; it consists of a soft rubber tube in the shape of a T, the transverse limb of which is placed in the duct while the vertical limb is brought out to the skin via a stab incision. The tube is left to drain into a bag for 10 days after surgery; if a stone has been left in the distal duct, the decompressive effect of the tube prevents leakage of bile into the peritoneum at the site of exploration. After 10 days, a T-tube cholangiogram is performed to exclude a retained stone; if all is well the tube is clamped for 24 hours and then simply pulled out. During the postoperative period, a track will have formed around the long limb of the tube, so that any transient leak of bile following tube removal passes harmlessly to the skin surface.

334 A mucocele of the gall-bladder occurs when the organ becomes distended with mucus; it develops when a gall-stone impacts in the cystic duct or Hartmann's pouch, preventing entry of bile or exit of gall-bladder mucus. If acute infection does

not supervene, producing an empyema, the gall-bladder mucosa will absorb the bile salts and pigments which will be carried away in the blood stream and replace them with mucus. The gall-bladder can become greatly distended and hence palpable below the right costal margin.

335 Bile duct strictures may be benign or malignant. More than 90% of benign strictures follow surgery on the biliary tract, while the remainder are due to other upper abdominal surgery, chronic pancreatitis or sclerosing cholangitis. Bile duct carcinoma is uncommon.

336 Although an uncommon disease, this is in fact the fifth most common digestive malignancy; it usually occurs in association with gall-stones. It spreads by local invasion of the liver and other surrounding organs, and to the local lymph nodes. The diagnosis is often first made at cholecystectomy for gall-stones; the tumour is usually unresectable, so that the prognosis is dismal — 80% are dead at 1 year, with a 5-year survival of less than 5%.

The spleen

337 The organs in particular danger are the pancreas, stomach and diaphragm. The pancreatic tail lies at the splenic hilum and can be damaged during ligation of the artery and vein; the upper part of the greater curve of the stomach is supplied by the short gastric branches of the splenic artery, so the stomach can be caught in the ties on these vessels; and the diaphragm may be adherent to the posterior surface of the spleen, in which case it can be pierced during initial mobilization. Other structures occasionally traumatized are the left kidney and adrenal gland and the splenic flexure of the colon.

338 The differences which may be detected on clinical examination are that it is possible to palpate above a kidney but not a spleen, a kidney moves up and down rather than obliquely across the abdomen, a notch may be palpated on a spleen but not a kidney, percussion over a kidney is usually resonant and a kidney can be balloted.

142

339   The commonest causes of splenomegaly in Europe are the myeloproliferative disorders, particularly myeloid leukaemia and Hodgkin's disease, portal hypertension due to cirrhosis, thrombocytopenic purpura and spherocytosis.

340   The usual indications for splenectomy are trauma, as a staging procedure in Hodgkin's disease, as a therapeutic measure in blood diseases such as thrombocytopenic purpura and spherocytosis and to correct hypersplenism in leukaemia or cirrhosis.

341   The early complications of splenectomy include haemorrhage from the splenic pedicle or splenic bed; venous thrombosis as a result of the greatly increased platelet count which may follow splenectomy; and fistula resulting from damage to the pancreas, stomach or colon. The important late complication is overwhelming sepsis, particularly in small children.

342   Splenomegaly means an enlarged spleen. If such an enlarged spleen starts sequestering white cells and platelets so that leucopenia and thrombocytopenia occur, the patient has hypersplenism. For example, splenomegaly due to portal hypertension may be followed by the development of hypersplenism.

The small bowel

343   The superior mesenteric artery supplies the small bowel. Having arisen from the aorta behind the pancreas, it passes downwards between the uncinate process and the neck of the pancreas to cross the third part of the duodenum, thus entering the root of the small bowel mesentery. Therein it runs downwards to the right towards its termination, about 15 cm proximal to the ileocaecal valve, crossing the vena cava, right psoas muscle and right ureter en route.

344   As the terminal ileum is the site of absorption of the intrinsic factor/vitamin B_{12} complex and the reabsorption of bile salts, there are two main consequences of its resection — first megaloblastic anaemia may develop when vitamin B_{12} stores be-

come depleted and second, depletion of the bile salt pool can lead to diarrhoea.

345 Most patients with small bowel Crohn's disease initially present with diarrhoea, colicky abdominal pain, malaise and weight loss. On examination there may be a mild pyrexia and in about 30% a mass may be felt, usually in the right iliac fossa. Around 10% of patients will have anal disease, fistula or fissure, even in the absence of other evidence of large bowel involvement with Crohn's disease.

346 The most important extra-abdominal manifestation of Crohn's disease is perianal sepsis — this may take the form of anal fissure (often multiple and with angry, oedematous surrounding skin) or fistula-in-ano, which may be complicated or accompanied by cavitation. Other such signs of Crohn's disease include oral aphthous ulceration, polyarthritis and erythema nodosum.

347 A barium follow-through examination will demonstrate several features in Crohn's disease. First there will be one or more segments of abnormality, usually in the distal small bowel — if there are more than one, they are known as skip lesions. Abnormal segments have a narrow, irregular lumen, with a thickened wall which holds other loops of bowel away, so that the narrowed segment stands out — the string sign of Kantor. Mucosal ulceration is usually visible, and there may be evidence of fistulae into other parts of the small or large bowel, into the bladder or occasionally on to the skin.

348 Surgery is undertaken for Crohn's disease in several circumstances; first in patients initially treated medically who fail to thrive, that is, remain unwell, underweight, anaemic and uncomfortable; second, surgery is indicated for the complications, particularly obstruction, fistula and abscess formation; finally it is sometimes necessary in order to contain the extra-abdominal manifestations of the disease, which usually improve once the diseased bowel is excised.

349 Intussusception describes the invagination of the proximal bowel into the distal bowel. In adults

there is usually an underlying lesion such as a lipoma, polyp or carcinoma which forms part of the intussusception. In infants there is often no immediately obvious cause and enlarged lymphoid aggregations have been blamed.

350 There are four ways in which Meckel's diverticulum can induce acute illness; it can become acutely inflamed — Meckel's diverticulitis — which precisely mimics acute appendicitis; it can cause small bowel obstruction by becoming adherent somewhere within the abdomen, often due to a fibrous band at its apex; it can perforate, usually at an ulcer arising at an island of ectopic gastric mucosa within it; or it can bleed from an ectopic peptic ulcer.

351 A patient with radiation damage to the bowel will present differently depending whether it is immediately after the radiation, within the first year or many years later. In the early period the patient may develop a perforation. Later the patient may develop an inflammatory mass of bowel causing a fistula or obstruction. After several years, radiation damage causes ischaemia leading to malabsorption and stricture formation.

352 There are three points about the fashioning of an ileostomy which deserve comment. First, its position — it is placed in the lower abdomen, away from the umbilicus, the anterior superior iliac spine, scars and the belt line so that the appliance fits nicely and is comfortable. Second, its spout shape — this is used so that the apex of the stoma lies well into the appliance to avoid skin maceration. Finally, the mucocutaneous suture — early ileostomies were simply spouts of bowel brought out through the skin, but the serosal surface often became fibrotic and contracted, leading to subacute obstruction. Simple doubling back of the bowel, and suture of the mucosa to the skin edge has largely overcome mechanical complications. Having an ileostomy can never be pleasant, but some cope better than others. It tends to produce liquid effluent continuously throughout the day and may overact if there is dietary indiscretion. It needs regular and careful maintenance to prevent skin damage. However, it need not prevent a full and active working and social life.

The peritoneal cavity

353 Ascites is diagnosed clinically by finding abdominal distension, a fluid thrill and shifting dullness. The first sign is non-specific and could otherwise be due to gaseous distension or a large mass, such as an ovarian cyst. A fluid thrill confirms the presence of a large volume of fluid and is elicited by flicking one side of the abdomen with the index finger and feeling the transmitted thrill with the other hand on the other side of the abdomen, while the edge of an assistant's hand presses on the centre of the abdomen to prevent transmission via the abdominal wall. The fact that the fluid is free within the peritoneum rather than in a cyst is confirmed by the shifting dullness test, in which the pattern of peripheral dullness and central resonance changes when the patient rolls 45° sideways, so that the gas in the intestine floats uppermost again. If doubt still exists, ultrasound examination can be performed. The major causes of ascites are malignancy, portal hypertension usually due to cirrhosis, right heart failure and the nephrotic syndrome.

354 The ascites can be drained to produce short-term relief, and chemotherapeutic agents instilled to try to prevent reaccumulation. This is best done, after making sure that the bladder is empty, by inserting a peritoneal dialysis cannula into the pelvis via the right iliac fossa or the linea alba under local anaesthesia. When all the fluid is drained, thiotepa, an alkylating agent, is injected via the cannula — the dose is 10 to 30 mg in 20 to 60 ml of sterile water; this can be repeated every 1 or 2 weeks if necessary.

355 Pelvic abscess is most commonly seen in patients who have already been treated for an intraperitoneal infective process, rather than in patients presenting de novo. The important initiating lesions are perforated appendicitis, perforated peptic ulcer and perforated diverticular disease. The symptoms suggestive of this condition are pelvic discomfort and diarrhoea, while on examination, there is a swinging fever and fullness of the pouch of Douglas, with induration of the overlying rectal wall. If necessary, the diagnosis is confirmed by ultrasound. Treatment is expectant

retrovesical pouch?

146

— the abscess usually drains spontaneously through the anterior rectal wall.

356 This accompanies 3–5% of mucinous ovarian tumours, and consists of gelatinous masses of mucin and tumour scattered through the peritoneal and abdominal cavities as a result of rupture of a mucinous cystadenoma. It may also arise from a mucocele of the appendix. Unfortunately despite removing this, the condition tends to keep recurring.

The large bowel

357 The colon as far as the distal transverse colon is supplied by branches of the superior mesenteric artery, i.e. the ileocolic, right colic and middle colic arteries. The colon from the splenic flexure distally, and the rectum, are supplied by the left colic, sigmoid and superior haemorrhoidal branches of the inferior mesenteric artery. The middle rectal branch of the internal iliac artery also contributes to the supply of the rectum.

358 The main point is that the longitudinal muscle of the colon is confined to the three taeniae coli, whereas it is spread evenly around the rectum. The blood vessels of the colon penetrate the wall vertically at the edges of the taeniae, producing potential 'channels' along which intraluminal pressure can, over a period, force the development of mucosal diverticula. However, the vessels supplying the rectum penetrate the wall more obliquely, so that luminal pressure does not force out diverticula alongside them.

359 The right ureter and kidney, the right testicular or ovarian vessels, the duodenum and pancreas.

360 The large bowel absorbs water and electrolytes from the material entering it from the ileum and acts as a reservoir for faecal matter until voiding is socially convenient. Of the 800 to 1000 ml of water presented to the large bowel each day, all but 150 ml is absorbed. Voiding of faeces is controlled by a complicated sensorimotor mechanism in which awareness of the presence of faeces in the rectum is mediated by nerve endings in the

bowel wall and pelvic floor; when the rectum is thus distended, a reflex relaxes the anal sphincter, though this can be voluntarily overridden if the time is not right for defaecation.

361   There is a lot of circumstantial evidence for a link between diet and colorectal cancer. The disease is rare in rural Africa and Asia, while those migrating from these areas to countries of high incidence are likely to develop the bowel cancer risk of their new home. This strongly suggests environmental risk factors, and diet is the most obvious. High levels of animal fat and low levels of dietary fibre are the most likely factors. Animal fat stimulates bile production, and bacterial breakdown of certain bile acids may produce cancer-promoting substances. Fibre probably has a protective effect by speeding colonic transit, and hence decreasing contact between mucosa and luminal cancer promoters. Some trace elements and vitamins — selenium, calcium, vitamins A and C — may act as 'chemopreventive' agents.

362   There are several rare, autosomal dominant conditions which predispose to colorectal cancer; in addition it is likely that there are many patients — perhaps more than 20% of those with the disease — in whom there is a polygenic predisposition. The rare dominant conditions include familial adenomatous polyposis (FAP) and the hereditary non-polyposis colorectal cancer syndromes (HNPCCS). In FAP colorectal adenomas appear around the mid-teens, some of which will progress to cancer in 15–20 years if preventive measures are not taken. Other abnormalities include upper gastro-intestinal adenomas, desmoid tumours, epidermoid and dental cysts, and retinal pigment spots. The gene for this condition is on the long arm of chromosome 5. There are two HNPCCSs — the Cancer Family Syndrome and the Site-Specific Colorectal Cancer Syndrome. Families exhibiting the latter develop large bowel tumours only, while in the former, ovarian, endometrial and other cancers occur. In these syndromes, cancers tend to occur earlier than average, there are more right-sided colon tumours, and more cases of second colorectal primaries. Four genes have been identified which may be responsible for these syndromes.

363 Screening is the search for disease in asymptomatic people. When used on a population-wide basis, it should be used only in common diseases in which it is known that earlier intervention will improve the outlook for the disease in the population. In the case of colorectal cancer, there is not yet sufficient evidence of its efficacy for national screening to have been set up in most countries. The most widely tested screening test is the faecal occult blood test (FOBT) which is capable of detecting blood shed in the faeces. The test has several major shortcomings — it misses 50% of cancers, it is positive in almost ten times as many subjects as actually have cancer, and many people are reluctant to do the test. Major controlled trials, involving tens of thousands of subjects, are being performed to measure the efficacy of FOBT screening. Other screening methods, for which there is less evidence of worth or which are at a very early stage of development, include the detection of 'cancer gene' products in the stool, and flexible sigmoidoscopy.

364 50% of all large bowel cancers occur in the rectum, a further 25% in the sigmoid colon and about 10% in the caecum. The remainder are spread fairly evenly throughout the rest of the colon.

365 Right-sided cancer classically presents with the symptoms of anaemia and debility, while left-sided lesions produce symptoms of advancing obstruction, that is, change of bowel habit and cramping abdominal pain, which may progress to frank obstruction. This difference occurs because the right colon is relatively wider and transmits a more liquid stool than the left colon (so that right-sided cancers can bleed and cause debility 'quietly'), while left-sided tumours tend to be the stricturing type, compared to the 'cauliflower' lesions which usually develop in the right colon.

366 One should start from the premise that the patient has cancer until proven otherwise, though other conditions, such as polyps, villous adenomas, diverticular disease and inflammatory bowel disease, can also produce these symptoms. After careful physical examination including digitation of the anus and proctosigmoidoscopy, a barium

enema is mandatory. If after clinical examination and radiology the diagnosis is not clear, colonoscopy should be performed.

367   As with most radical operations for cancer, large bowel procedures comprise removal of the primary lesion together with its lymphatic draining in the hope that this will achieve removal of all malignant tissue. As the nodes and lymphatics draining the colon and rectum lie along the arteries to the bowel, the relevant arteries are traced to their source, and flush-tied, followed by their removal with the involved segment of bowel.

368   This is a system of pathological staging applied to operative specimens and has been shown to provide the most precise prognostic information available at the time of primary treatment. The Dukes' system describes Stage A, in which there is spread of growth into the submucosa or muscle but not beyond, and with no lymph node involvement; Stage B, when the tumour penetrates through bowel wall without node involvement; and Stage C in which whatever the spread within or through the bowel wall, lymph nodes are involved. Over 90% of Stage A patients can expect to survive at least 5 years while for Stages B and C, the corresponding figures are about 60% and 30% respectively.

369   Ulcerative colitis, familial adenomatous polyposis and simple adenomatous polyps. The risk of malignancy in ulcerative colitis is especially important in those with total colitis and among those in whom the disease developed at a young age. If these two criteria are present, the risk of cancer having developed within 25 years of the onset of colitis is up to 13%. In those with familial adenomatous polyposis, in which the large bowel mucosa becomes covered by thousands of polyps, malignancy will always supervene if prophylactic colectomy is not performed. As far as simple adenomatous polyps are concerned, there is evidence that most carcinomas arise from these lesions, though most polyps do not progress to malignancy.

370   Thrombo-embolic conditions may interfere with the blood supply of the large bowel, particularly the colon. The commonest lesion is arterial embolism, usually secondary to atrial fibrillation

150

or myocardial infarction. Most commonly an embolus enters the superior mesenteric artery (SMA), when the ischaemic injury may include the right colon. Arterial thrombosis may involve the inferior mesenteric artery, producing a variable segment of large bowel ischaemia. Collateral flow from the SMA and the rectal arterial supply from the iliac arteries may prevent generalized critical ischaemia — in this situation, this may be confined to the region of the splenic flexure. Depending on the degree of ischaemia caused, the injury may range from mucosal oedema and haemorrhage, manifesting as diarrhoea and rectal bleeding, to systemic collapse, septicaemia and peritonitis due to full thickness infarction of the affected segment.

371 Although the theory is by no means proven, it is commonly believed that the initial problem lies in the low fibre content of the Western diet. This leads to low volume, firm stools, the passage of which is difficult, leading to colonic muscular hypertrophy, greatly raised intraluminal pressure and finally the forcing out of mucosal diverticula next to the blood vessels piercing the bowel wall along the edges of the taeniae coli. Colonic diverticular disease is very common. Although usually asymptomatic, it can be shown radiologically that one-third of the population have this condition at the age of 60 and two-thirds at 80.

372 Most commonly, diverticular disease presents with flatulence, a sensation of bloating and lower abdominal pain or discomfort. The bowel function is variable, but often with a tendency to pass small, pellet-like stools. If pain is present it is usually described as like 'wind pain', and may be mainly in the left iliac fossa. All these symptoms are presumed to be due to activity of the hypertrophic colonic muscle.

373 First, the nature of diverticular disease should be explained to him, indicating the need to increase the roughage content of the diet with the aims of eradicating present symptoms and preventing future complications. Then he should be given instructions regarding a high fibre diet and asked to use this as part of his daily routine in future. The instructions include the use of unprocessed bran (mixed with the breakfast cereal) and wholemeal

bread and the regular intake of fruit and vegetables.

374   Acute diverticulitis; pericolic abscess; peritonitis, either faecal due to perforation of a diverticulum or purulent due to rupture of a pericolic abscess; haemorrhage; fistula formation; and obstruction. All develop due to infection or erosion around diverticula. Infection occurs readily in the narrow-necked diverticula, leading on to a generalized inflammatory process (diverticulitis) which unusually may cause obstruction of the lumen of the bowel. Suppuration in an inflamed area leads to a pericolic abscess, which can rupture into the peritoneum or into a nearby organ, particularly the bladder, producing a fistula. Finally erosion at the neck of a diverticulum can lead to perforation or haemorrhage from the blood vessels next to it.

375   The important diagnosis that may not have been excluded is colonic cancer, as the muscle hypertrophy induced by the diverticular disease can make the spotting of a malignant stricture difficult. If the surgeon or radiologist is unhappy, a colonoscopy should be performed as this is the only investigation that can properly exclude malignancy.

376   There are two types of rectal prolapse — incomplete, in which only the mucosa protrudes, and complete, in which the whole thickness of the rectal wall prolapses, constituting an intussusception of the distal bowel through a weakened pelvic floor. Incomplete (mucosal) prolapse can occur at any age, while complete prolapse occurs mainly in young children and old ladies, especially those who have a long history of straining at stool.

377   Surgery offers the only possibility of cure in this age group. The commonest and most satisfactory procedure is the Ivalon rectopexy, in which, via an abdominal approach, the rectum is fully mobilized, a sheet of Ivalon sponge is placed into the sacral concavity and the rectum sutured to it; subsequent fibrosis prevents prolapse. Other procedures are less satisfactory — anterior resection is more risky while the more minor Thiersch operation, in which a wire or nylon suture is placed around the anus, usually leads to faecal impaction and often fails ultimately due to

breakage of the suture. Delorme's operation, mucosal excision and muscle plication, is an alternative perineal procedure.

378 The complications of ulcerative colitis can be divided into local and systemic. Local complications include toxic megacolon, perforation, massive haemorrhage, benign stricture and carcinoma. The first two require urgent surgery, while haemorrhage alone rarely leads to operation. Benign strictures develop in about 10% of patients with chronic disease and must be differentiated from cancer. Malignant changes occur mainly in those with total colitis and a long history, and in whom the initial attack was severe. Systemic complications, most of which are uncommon or rare, include arthritis, especially ankylosing spondylitis; skin conditions such as erythema nodosum and pyoderma gangrenosum; eye lesions — iritis and episcleritis; and hepatobiliary problems such as cirrhosis, sclerosing cholangitis and bile duct carcinoma.

379 There are emergency, urgent and elective indications for surgery in ulcerative colitis. The emergency indications are the acute complications — perforation, toxic megacolon and continuing massive haemorrhage. Surgery is required urgently in the fulminating case not responding to several days of aggressive medical treatment, while elective surgery is required for carcinoma, severe dysplasia (indicating imminent malignant change), chronic debility or stunted growth in the pubertal patient. The usual elective procedures are ileoanal pouch or proctocolectomy with ileostomy. In emergencies, or if the rectum is relatively mildly affected, the rectum may be left in situ, the proximal end being brought out as a mucus fistula; later an ileorectal anastomosis or ileal pouch may be fashioned, or the rectum excised with or without pouch formation.

380 Crohn's disease affects the large bowel in about one-third of patients, either alone or in combination with small bowel disease. When Crohn's disease affects the large bowel it produces symptoms akin to ulcerative colitis, that is, diarrhoea and bleeding, often with weight loss and general debility. Very commonly it affects the anus, producing fissures which may be multiple, abscesses and complex fistulae.

381 Drugs used in the treatment of ulcerative colitis include salicylate-based drugs, steroids and immunosuppressive agents. Salicylate-based drugs may be taken either orally or by enema — they include salazopyrine, mesalazine and olsalazine. They are particularly useful in maintaining remission once this has occurred spontaneously, sometimes after initial use of steroids. Steroids — most commonly prednisolone — are used primarily to arrest acute exacerbations. They can be given topically as suppositories or enemas, orally or intravenously. Their systemic use should be limited to restrict the risk of side effects. Immunosuppressive agents include azathioprine, cyclosporine and 6-mercaptopurine. These are used as second line drugs in those patients in whom steroids have not induced remission, or in whom oral steroids are contra-indicated or need to be curtailed after prolonged use. All of these medications are used in Crohn's disease, but in general they are less effective.

382 No — most patients settle on bed rest and blood transfusion. If haemorrhage continues or recurs, surgery must be considered; selective arteriography is the investigation of choice to locate the site of haemorrhage so that the appropriate bowel segment can be resected. Barium studies and endoscopy rarely locate the site of active haemorrhage particularly if this is due to angiodysplasia.

383 The most likely cause for this clinical picture is the irritable bowel syndrome. This is an ill-understood condition which is assumed to be due to functional disorder of the large, and perhaps also the small, intestine. There are no specific confirmatory tests so the diagnosis is made usually after exclusion by appropriate investigation of other conditions with similar symptoms, particularly Crohn's disease in this case. In older patients — those in their 50s and onwards — it is particularly important to be sure that more serious conditions, especially bowel cancer, are not responsible for the symptoms before making this diagnosis.

384 Colorectal polyps, usually adenomas, are not often symptomatic. The commonest symptom is bleeding on defaecation. Mucus discharge, particularly from rectal polyps and especially large

villous lesions, may occur. Rarely, mucus loss from a rectal villous adenoma can cause hypo-kalaemia, which may induce lethargy, fainting and cardiac dysrhythmias. Distal rectal polyps may prolapse through the anus, and be mistaken for piles. Most colorectal polyps can be removed via an endoscope, usually using biopsy forceps or by 'lassooing' them using a wire snare through which an electric cutting current is passed. Sometimes surgery is required for larger polyps particularly those with a broad base; rectal lesions may be removed transanally, while endoscopically un-resectable colonic lesions may require segmental resection.

The anus and anal canal

385 Puborectalis, the upper part of the external anal sphincter, is vital for faecal continence. The rest of the external sphincter and the internal sphincter can be divided, as for example, in fistula surgery; such extensive division may produce incontinence of flatus or of very loose stool, but normal stool can be controlled so long as puborectalis remains intact.

386 The lower half of the anal canal is lined by squamous epithelium, while the rest is lined by rectal-type mucosa. The distal part of the skin-covered area contains glands and has hair. The transition between the skin and mucosa occurs at the dentate line, which is often very tortuous with islands of either cell type to be found above and below the line.

387 In the UK, this examination is usually performed with the patient lying in the left lateral position, although in some parts of the world the knee-elbow position is used. After explaining gently to the patient what is about to happen, the lubri-cated, gloved right index finger is placed at the anus and gently introduced into the anal canal. At this early stage the resting tone of the sphincters can be assessed; by use of the thumb externally and the finger within, the sphincters and sur-rounding tissues can be palpated bidigitally to assess the integrity of the sphincter ring and to look for induration due to sepsis or tumour. The finger is then inserted further, allowing palpation

of the prostate gland, and then of the lower rectum and surrounding tissues. When the finger is withdrawn, it should be examined looking at the nature of the stool and for the presence of blood or mucus.

388 The commonest symptom is bleeding on defaecation, usually first noted as blood on the toilet paper. Other symptoms include discomfort after defaecation, pruritis ani and prolapse which may or may not require manual reduction. Pain is unusual, except when piles become strangulated, or if another lesion, such as a fissure, is co-existent.

389 Many patients make a self-diagnosis of piles if they pass blood. The doctor must never omit digital examination and proctosigmoidoscopy to exclude more serious causes of bleeding — this usually requires referral to hospital. Unless the symptoms and endoscopic findings all point towards piles as the cause of bleeding, and especially in the over 40s, it is best to perform a barium enema — change of bowel habit, passage of mucus, abdominal pain, weight loss, the finding of free mucus in the rectum all demand this investigation. In short, piles are so common that a possible co-existing lesion higher in the bowel must always be energetically excluded if clinical findings suggest the need.

390 There are three degrees of piles — first-degree piles cause symptoms, usually bleeding but do not prolapse; second-degree piles prolapse but reduce spontaneously; while third-degree piles prolapse and require manual reduction. First-degree piles are best treated by sclerosant injection, and correction of any constipation with a high fibre diet. Second-degree piles can be treated either by injection or by the use of the elastic banding technique, while third-degree piles can be banded if small enough, or removed by haemorrhoidectomy if large, especially if there are accompanying skin tags. Today only 5% of pile patients require haemorrhoidectomy.

391 I would remember that this is called reactionary haemorrhage and that it may be due to minor ooze from the cut surface which should respond

to conservative measures, but can also be a major bleed from a single vessel which will require further surgery to stop it. Having checked the vital signs and seen the extent of the external bleeding, I would elevate the foot of the bed which may 'take the pressure off the piles', calm the patient, using sedation if necessary, take blood for cross-match and put up a drip if the bleed seems serious. I would alert my senior colleagues, who would decide to return to theatre if the haemorrhage were large or persistent.

392 An anal fissure is a longitudinal ulcer, usually in the posterior midline of the distal anal canal and is often, though not exclusively, associated with constipation and sphincter spasm. The patient gives a history of variable length, most often complaining of pain and bleeding on defaecation, perhaps with pruritis or a discharge; the bleeding is usually only noticed on wiping. On examination, a sentinel skin tag and the lower part of the fissure may be seen on gently parting the buttocks. Gentle digital examination may reveal sphincter spasm and induration around the fissure. If proctoscopy is not too painful to perform, it will demonstrate the length of the fissure, perhaps with the internal sphincter visible in its base and a proximal fibrous anal polyp if present.

393 A fistula-in-ano is an abnormal communication between the anal canal (or rarely the lower rectum) and the perianal skin. It arises following an infection in one of the anal glands, which open into the anal canal at the dentate line and which ramify in the space between the internal and external sphincters. The infection may spread down this intersphincteric space or through the external sphincter into the ischiorectal fossa, either way then bursting through on to the perianal skin. Thus the majority of fistulae open internally at the dentate line (via the anal gland in which the infection started), while the site of the external opening is variable. Other ramifications are less common. The diagnosis is based on a history of continuous or intermittent perianal discharge, perhaps with occasional abscess formation, and the finding of an external opening on the perianal skin and an internal opening in the canal — the latter is sometimes only confirmed at operation.

394 Anal fistulae can only be treated surgically. At operation, the first aim is to define the anatomy of the lesion accurately using probes. Next the track is laid open by dividing all tissue superficial to it by cutting down on to a probe in the fistula; the wound is then lightly dressed. Treatment continues on the ward, with once or twice daily baths, irrigation and light redressing of the cavity, aiming to induce healing in the deeper part of the wound first. The major danger of operation is that the surgeon may not recognize that a high fistula passes through or even above puborectalis — if he then divides all tissue superficial to the track, he would divide the sphincter, causing faecal incontinence.

395 The most common disease causing perianal sepsis is Crohn's disease. Others include tuberculosis, the human immunodeficiency virus (HIV) and leukaemia, the latter two sometimes causing particularly extensive and troublesome lesions.

396 Having excluded faecal impaction, rectal prolapse and senility, most cases of faecal incontinence in women are due to damage caused during childbirth. This may involve direct tearing due to the size of the baby or use of forceps, or accidental cutting of the sphincters during episiotomy; often there is traction injury to the pudendal nerves which supply the external sphincter, leading to lowered squeeze pressure. In some women, as in men, incontinence may be due to other causes, including anal surgery — especially for fistula — and trauma.

397 Choice of treatment comes after careful assessment, including establishment of the most likely cause and investigation to differentiate discrete sphincter injury from pudendal neuropathy. In cases of minor incontinence, measures to make the stool firmer and less frequent may help; dietary manipulation and mild constipating agents may help in this way. In more serious cases, surgery to repair the defect or to tighten a slack neuropathic sphincter may be required. Repair of an isolated sphincter injury is usually very helpful in an otherwise healthy patient with an otherwise normal sphincter.

398   All types of anal malignancy are uncommon, but the lesions most frequently encountered are squamous cell carcinoma and basaloid carcinoma. Adenocarcinoma can arise above the dentate line, while melanoma also usually arises high in the canal. While adenocarcinoma spreads to the abdominal nodes, like rectal cancer, the other tumours spread first to the lymph nodes in the groin.

399   The most important STDs to involve the anus are those associated with human papilloma virus (HPV) infection, AIDS lesions, and syphilis. HPV infection is very common, usually manifesting as anal warts. Much less common is anal carcinoma, a majority of cases of which are probably due to oncogenic HPV types. AIDS may cause various anal lesions, typically perianal sepsis or ulceration; Kaposi's sarcoma can occur in the anus and rectum, producing purple patches which could be mis-diagnosed as piles. Primary syphilis may produce anal sores which may be mistaken for fissure or Crohn's disease. Secondary syphilis manifests as perianal dermatitis or condylomata lata, reddened hypertrophic papules which are clinically distinguishable from condy-lomata acuminatum (viral warts). Other STDs which may affect the anus are granuloma venereum and lymphogranuloma inguinale.

400   This is the term applied to a localized area of thrombosis in the veins beneath the perianal skin; it is otherwise known as a thrombosed external haemorrhoid. It presents as a severely painful perianal lump, which may be small, spherical and blue or rather more diffuse and lighter in colour. It is initially very tender, but this usually eases after several days.

THE BREAST

401   Lymph from the breast drains medially and laterally. The medial half of the breast drains predominantly to the nodes situated along the internal mammary artery, which runs behind the anterior ends of the ribs; the lateral half of the breast drains to the axillary nodes, which lie along the

medial axillary wall from the tail of the breast to the apex of the axilla.

402 If the nipple discharge is clear or milky, bilateral, appears on massaging the breast or nipple and there is no lump to feel in the breast, then the discharge is more likely to be physiological in origin. By contrast, a spontaneous, unilateral blood stained discharge is more likely to be related to an underlying duct papilloma, duct ectasia and sometimes a breast carcinoma.

403 The two symptoms may be unconnected. However, malignant pleural effusion occurs in 50% of patients with breast carcinoma at some stage of the illness; the possibility that the lump is malignant and that the patient has a pleural effusion must be seriously considered.

404 A malignant breast lump may produce deformity of the affected breast, dimpling of the overlying skin, inversion of the nipple or peau d'orange; sometimes skin ulceration may be present. Breast cancers are very variable in size, so this factor does not aid differential diagnosis. The edges of a malignant breast lump are usually ill-defined, the surface irregular and the consistency very firm. With more advanced lesions fixity to skin and pectoral muscles may be detected.

405 Both of these physical signs strongly suggest that a breast lump is malignant. Tethering is due to malignant involvement of the fibrous bands (ligaments of Astley-Cooper) which connect the skin of the breast to the pectoral fascia; it produces dimpling or decreased mobility of the skin overlying the lump, but some mobility is maintained. Fixity implies direct spread of the malignancy into the skin, preventing any 'sliding' of the skin over the lump by the examining hand. Fixity is a sign of locally advanced disease, while tethering, of itself, carries no prognostic significance.

406 This is a presentation of breast cancer sometimes seen in the elderly. The patient often has no idea of the length of the history and may be totally unperturbed by the lesion. The cancer causes the breast to contract markedly so that sometimes no normal tissue remains. The scab represents an area of ulceration. Although these lesions are

obviously locally advanced, there is frequently no evidence of spread beyond the chest wall. The majority of such cases respond well to oestrogens, oestrogen antagonists or local radiotherapy, preventing the development of distressing symptoms.

407   The recent development of unilateral nipple inversion must be regarded as due to the presence of breast cancer until proven otherwise. If, as is usual, a lump cannot be felt deep to a recently inverted nipple, further investigation including mammography is mandatory to locate the causative lesion. Long-standing inversion, unilateral or bilateral, has no sinister significance.

408   This is a condition in which the nipple develops an appearance identical to eczema; it is due to the development of an intraduct carcinoma which may, or may not, be palpable. Histology reveals the presence of large vacuolated cells with small, dark nuclei in the epidermis. This condition must be differentiated from true, simple eczema which is always bilateral and has no malignant association. When Paget's disease of the nipple is diagnosed, carcinoma can be assumed and managed accordingly.

409   This is a physical sign usually associated with breast cancer, but sometimes seen with a breast abscess. The skin overlying the lesion literally takes on the appearance of orange peel; it is due to lymphatic oedema caused by the underlying disease.

410   This is due to lymphoedema, which occurs when the axillary nodes become damaged or destroyed by the presence of secondary growth, by radiotherapy or by surgical removal in radical mastectomy. The arm becomes swollen, sometimes enormously, making it heavy and difficult to use. Rarely, it causes lymphosarcoma. Lymphoedema occurs in about 5 to 10% of patients who have had radiotherapy or radical surgery.

411   Mammography of the breasts is the standard screening method where it is used particularly to look for microcalcification within the breast. It can help in determining whether a lump is a carcinoma or benign, but it is not completely reliable in this regard so that suspicious breast lumps

need removal whatever the mammogram results. Mammography is good at demonstrating multi-focal ductal carcinoma in situ (DCIS) and so may indicate those patients who require a mastectomy rather than a lumpectomy. Where a small impalpable lesion is demonstrated at mammography, guide wire localization may be required under mammographic imaging to determine the site for biopsy excision.

412 A lesion with a spiculated, ill-defined margin on mammography is almost certainly a breast cancer unless the patient has had previous surgery at the site. Microcalcification, particularly when grouped in clusters within a particular area, is very suggestive of underlying malignancy although fine needle aspiration cytology is required to confirm this. Other radiological changes such as asymmetry of breast architecture are less clear cut.

413 Breast cancer screening is of proven benefit for patients aged 50–75 years. It is also probably of value to patients aged 40–50 who have a strong family history for the disease. Below this age, the mammographic changes of breast cancer are difficult to identify against the background of the healthy breast tissue. Screening is based on mammography but may also be based on patient self-examination and clinical examinations; neither of these methods is of proven benefit in terms of cancer survival.

414 Radiology helps us to assess the primary lesion and to look for secondary spread. In women under 35, ultrasound is the preferred method of assessment of breast lumps since the breasts are difficult to assess by mammography in young women. For women over 35 mammography is preferred, looking particularly for microcalcification and other densities within the breasts. Mammography and ultrasound can be used to direct localization and fine needle aspiration cytology of breast lumps.

415 The state of the axillary nodes is the single most important factor in assessing prognosis in breast cancer. Ten years after primary treatment, around two-thirds of patients whose axillary nodes were

free of disease will still be alive, compared to one-third if there was nodal spread.

416   The commonest sites for distant spread are bone, liver, lungs and pleura, in that order.

417   For many years, it was assumed that breast cancer spread in stepwise fashion, that is, that the primary enlarged, followed by lymph node involvement and finally generalized, blood-borne dissemination. More recently it has been suggested that widespread occult micrometastases may occur at an extremely early stage and that the appearance, or not, of obvious dissemination reflects host response to the tumour. The first of these theories resulted in the concept that 'the more radical the operation, the greater the chance of cure'. However, radical local surgery has not affected the incidence of distant spread. This has lent support to the theory of early occult metastases and has resulted in a more conservative surgical approach to the primary disease.

418   If an area of microcalcification is impalpable but is associated with an abnormal cytology, then the patient is taken down to mammography where the area is localized by compressing the area in a plastic grid and screening, in two dimensions, the breast on X-ray. The radiologist then passes a guide wire through a needle to as close as possible to the site. The patient comes down to theatre with the wire taped to the skin. Under general anaesthetic, the surgeon passes a needle over the wire to aid palpation and then makes a separate cut down to the tip of the wire which is excised to include the area of microcalcification. Before removal of the lump, sutures are inserted to help the pathologist with orientation of the specimen. The specimen is X-rayed to check that the area has been adequately excised prior to waking the patient.

419   Patients with large breast tumours and small breasts will usually have a poor cosmetic result with local excision of a breast tumour. Patients found to have extensive ductal carcinoma in situ in addition to a carcinoma, will also require a mastectomy to prevent recurrence. Paget's disease of the nipple is treated by mastectomy.

Finally patients unwilling or unable to have radio-therapy are better advised to have a mastectomy because of the high incidence of local recurrence following lumpectomy alone.

420 Simple mastectomy is an operation in which the whole of one breast, and no other tissue, is removed. Radical mastectomy involves the removal of a breast, together with its axillary lymphatic field. Complete node clearance requires removal of one or both of the pectoral muscles, to allow access to the apex of the axilla. In the 'classical' radical mastectomy the breast, nodes and both pectoral muscles are taken en bloc, while the 'modified' or 'Patey' radical procedures leaves the pectoralis major intact.

421 Surgeons and radiotherapists around the country differ in their attitudes to extent of surgery and the use of radiotherapy in the potentially curable case. However, on the basis of controlled trials, radiotherapy has been shown to have no effect on survival, but to decrease the incidence of local recurrence, especially in patients who have undergone lumpectomy. A full axillary dissection of lymph nodes followed by radiotherapy can induce lymphoedema. Hence some surgeons prefer only to irradiate axillas which have not been extensively dissected.

422 The patient is usually fitted with an external prosthesis, though several surgical replacements are also possible. Normally the patient wears a light, temporary prosthesis in her bra for the first 6 weeks, and later can choose from a variety of devices, either of soft foam or filled with liquid silicone or glycerine to mimic the normal texture. In some circumstances, a breast reconstruction, to build an internal replacement of the breast, using a prosthesis or muscle or omental grafts, can be performed, sometimes simultaneously with the mastectomy but more commonly 1 or 2 years after mastectomy.

423 There are four main patterns. First, some tumours become locally advanced, with no evidence of distant spread; typically this group is represented by the ulcerating scirrhous lesion in an old lady. Second, a patient may present with an apparently 'early' primary, but be found on inves-

164

tigation to have distant spread. Third, distant spread or local recurrence may develop after previous radical treatment of an 'early' primary tumour. Fourth, a patient may present with symptoms due to distant disease, such as bone pain, and be found on examination to have a small, previously unnoticed breast primary. Each of these situations will require a different management approach.

424 Two sorts of surgery can be considered in the treatment of advanced breast cancer — surgery to the primary and various endocrine ablative procedures. Removal of the primary tumour, if not 'locally advanced', is usually performed in patients with distant spread to prevent distressing progression of disease on the chest wall; the usual operation would be simple mastectomy. Endocrine ablative procedures, oophorectomy, hypophysectomy and adrenalectomy — which frequently produce remissions in advanced cases — have been largely superseded by medical ablative treatment.

425 Pain is the major mode of presentation for bone metastases — about half of all patients with distant spread in breast cancer require treatment for this problem. The other major mode of presentation is pathological fracture — commonest sites are in the vertebral column, sometimes causing paraplegia and in the femur. Pain from bone secondaries is usually rapidly relieved by irradiation. Early mobilization is important after fractures, as these patients have a short prognosis, so femoral fractures are best pinned and irradiated. Spinal lesions are sometimes an indication for laminectomy to try to alleviate or prevent spinal cord compression.

426 There are two forms of endocrine manipulation in advanced breast cancer — medical and surgical. Medical techniques include administration of oestrogens, tamoxifen (an oestrogen receptor antagonist), LHRH agonists such as Zoladex, progestogens such as megesterol, androgens such as fluoxymesterone and the adrenal steroid synthesis inhibitor, aminoglutethimide. Surgical procedures comprise oophorectomy, hypophysectomy and adrenalectomy although the latter two are rarely used now. The first choice in

premenopausal women is still probably oophorectomy, although this is controversial, while in
the postmenopausal, oestrogen or tamoxifen
therapy are first-line approaches. Major endocrine ablation has been superseded by aminoglutethimide, which should be reserved for use in
relapse following successful first-line treatment.
Remission occurs in about 30% of patients in
response to endocrine therapy and more frequently if oestrogen receptors are present in the
primary tumour.

427　The lifetime risk of developing a second breast
cancer in the other breast is about 10%. The risk
is about 1% per year of follow-up and is about five
times the risk for the general population. Because
of these figures, annual mammographic screening
of the other breast is recommended as well as
regular examination at follow-up in surgical outpatients.

428　A breast mouse is a fibro-adenoma. This term was
coined at some time in the past to characterize the
mobility of the lesion — it seems to run away and
hide when touched by the examining hand.

429　A cyst is usually ovoid, firm, fairly discrete and
smooth; it is not as mobile as a fibro-adenoma.
Unlike other cysts, lesions in the breast cannot be
tested for fluctuance or transillumination as they
are deeply placed. The most important confirmatory physical sign is successful, complete aspiration of fluid so that the lesion disappears.

430　Generalized lumpiness is usually due to benign
breast change (also referred to as fibro-adenosis,
fibrocystic disease, sclerosing adenosis or chronic
mastitis). This condition occurs most commonly
in multiparous women, especially towards the
menopause. Usually a segment of the breast is
involved, while sometimes the area is small, mimicking cancer by its vague outline and its irregularity. Benign breast change is not dangerous and
is best left alone, but any question of cancer in a
small nodular area must be resolved by open
biopsy.

431　The cardinal clinical feature is discharge from the
nipple which is either bloody or brown. Palpation
will often reveal a small lump deep to the areola,

pressure upon which produces further discharge from the nipple, confined to the opening from the relevant duct.

432   A 2 ml syringe and 20 gauge needle may be held in the hand or with a special holder. The lump is then located and held in the opposite hand whilst the skin is wiped and the needle inserted. The needle is moved vigorously through the lump whilst pulling on the plunger so as to encourage harvesting of cells without causing haemorrhage. The plunger is released and the needle withdrawn. The needle is removed from the syringe, the plunger pulled back and the needle then replaced so that the cells can be squirted out on to the slide. The cells are smeared with the second slide and immediately fixed. The value of this examination is that it may avoid the need for excision biopsy in some cases.

433   The residual lump should be removed. Although it is likely that it is due to benign fibrocystic disease, a carcinoma may be present, so excision biopsy is necessary to exclude this.

434   Careful questioning will usually reveal that the pain occurs around period time — such pain is thought to be related to changes in hormone levels associated with menstruation and is termed cyclical mastalgia. So long as no discrete lump is present, the woman should be reassured straight away that she does not have cancer. Evening primrose oil will help some patients if taken for several months. But if persistent and severe, the pain may be relieved by danazol, a synthetic progestin, or by bromocriptine, which affects prolactin production. But both drugs may induce side effects which discourage their widespread use in the treatment of mastalgia.

435   There are two histological patterns in fibroadenoma, the pericanalicular and the intracanalicular; both have a well-defined capsule, and both have an epithelial element in a fibrous tissue stroma. In the pericanalicular lesion, the epithelium forms ductules within the fibrous tissue, while the intracanalicular fibro-adenoma comprises fibrous tissue projecting into the duct system, which is thus stretched over it as a single layer of cells.

436   Fat necrosis, which occurs after trauma to the breast, can mimic carcinoma of the breast. It presents as an irregular, ill-defined breast lump, sometimes with skin tethering. A history of trauma does not exclude cancer, as many women ascribe breast tumours to this cause. Excision biopsy is mandatory. Bloody nipple discharge, often thought to be a sign of intraduct carcinoma is in fact usually due to benign papilloma; again, histology must be sought. Nipple inversion may suggest malignancy but if it is long-standing, and especially if bilateral, it is innocent. Nipple eczema can mimic Paget's disease of the nipple but is always bilateral. Finally, Mondor's disease, thrombophlebitis of the superficial veins of the breast, can mimic carcinoma.

437   Breast abscesses occur most commonly in breast feeding mothers, in whom the milk forms the perfect culture medium. However, this condition can occur in non-lactating young women. Occasionally neonates lactate under the influence of transplacental maternal prolactin, so they occasionally develop breast abscesses. Finally this lesion can occur in menopausal women in whom hormone fluctuations lead to secretions which can become infected.

438   A segment of the breast becomes painful and throbbing. On examination, there is erythema, perhaps peau d'orange, induration and tenderness in the affected area. These signs are sufficient indication for surgery. Fluctuation is a late sign in breast abscess and should not be awaited.

439   The lump represents a blocked segment of the breast which predisposes to bacterial mastitis and which can progress to an abscess if not treated. After examining her to confirm the diagnosis you would encourage her to go on feeding from both breasts whilst reassuring her that the baby will not become infected. If she developed a temperature, she might need flucloxacillin because of a staphylococcal infection. Rarely she might progress to an abscess requiring surgical drainage.

440   As with all abscesses, a breast abscess needs adequate incision and drainage. This entails incision over the apparent centre of the lesion

(fluctuation is not usually present to guide the surgeon), digital breakdown of loculi, despatch of pus for culture and light dressing of the cavity to prevent premature closure. Antibiotics and inhibition of lactation are not normally required. Recurrent abscesses in non-lactating women may necessitate microdochectomy. The usual organism is *Staphylococcus*, which may infect the breast by passage from the nasopharynx of the suckling infant.

441 Cyclical mastalgia is pain in the breasts which comes before menstruation each month. It is a difficult problem because of the poor response to treatment. Improvement has been reported with evening primrose oil, danazol, bromocriptine, pyridoxine (vitamin B_6) and the contraceptive pill.

442 This term literally means 'female breast' and refers to the condition in which breast tissue develops abnormally in the male. This happens frequently at puberty, usually resolving spontaneously; it can also develop in other situations in which hormone imbalance occurs, including cirrhosis (impaired clearance of hormones from the blood), stilboestrol therapy for prostatic cancer and the abnormality of sex chromosomes, Klinefelter's syndrome. Treatment is only required in patients in whom it persists, causing embarrassment — subareolar excision of the breast disc is the procedure used.

443 A plastic surgeon may operate on the breast to alter its size or to reconstruct it following mastectomy. Breast augmentation can be performed in women whose natural breasts are very small — the usual technique is the submammary placement of an appropriately sized plastic sac containing liquid silicone. A similar technique or a procedure involving the incorporation of a pedicle graft of omentum or latissimus dorsi can be used to replace a breast after mastectomy. Breast reduction, in which massive breasts are decreased to normal size, retaining the nipple, is indicated in young women who have abnormally large pendulous breasts which have proven uncomfortable and unattractive.

THE ENDOCRINE SYSTEM

444 The thyroid develops from the median bud of the pharynx and descends from the base of the tongue to its position in the neck. Arrest of descent can occur at any point. A lingual thyroid is found at the base of the tongue and may be the only functioning thyroid tissue present. A median ectopic thyroid is found as a midline swelling in the upper part of the neck. A thyroglossal cyst can form anywhere along the line of normal thyroid descent. Sometimes the cyst can become infected and rupture, forming a so-called thyroglossal fistula.

445 Inorganic iodide is taken up by the gland, oxidized to iodine and bound to tyrosine to form either mono- or di-iodotyrosine which combine to form T3 (tri-iodothyronine) and T4 (thyroxine).

446 The serum levels of T3 and T4 are measured by radio-immunoassay. The T3 uptake test is a measure of the capacity of iodine binding sites and when used in combination with serum T4 levels gives a value for the free thyroxine index (FTI = T4/T3 uptake × 100). Thyroid-stimulating hormone (TSH) can be measured by radio-immunoassay and is most useful in the diagnosis of hypothyroidism. Thyroid scanning with I^{131} or Technetium^{99} will reveal areas of functioning or non-functioning thyroid tissue.

447 This indicates an area of low or non-function, usually due to a cyst or a colloid nodule, but in about 12% of cases it represents a neoplasm. A cold nodule should therefore be viewed with suspicion and explored surgically, or if cystic, perhaps aspirated under ultrasound control.

448 A non-toxic goitre may be caused by an inadequate amount of iodine in the diet as may occur in mountainous areas where it is sometimes endemic. It can also be due to a congenital defect in the enzymes responsible for the uptake and utilization of iodide, or the presence of substances in the diet capable of blocking the uptake of iodide, such as thiocyanate which is found in vegetables of the brassica family. A non-toxic goitre may also result from autoimmune thyroiditis, carcinoma or

170

from cystic degeneration of the thyroid as seen in a multinodular goitre.

449 Cysts of the thyroid can be cured by aspiration alone. Anaplastic carcinoma can be accurately diagnosed and treated by radiotherapy. Cytology is less accurate at diagnosing papillary and follicular carcinomas and it is therefore not so valuable in the management of solitary nodules in the gland.

450 Thyrotoxicosis may be due to a primary overactivity of the gland which becomes uniformly enlarged and vascular (Graves' disease), toxic transformation in a long-standing nodular goitre, or occasionally from a solitary autonomous adenoma in the gland. Rarely, overdose with thyroxine replacement may produce symptoms and signs of thyrotoxicosis.

451 The patient is anxious and irritable. There may be a history of weight loss, diarrhoea, polydipsia and intolerance of hot weather. On examination, there is tachycardia, sometimes atrial fibrillation, exophthalmos, tremor and increased sweating; the thyroid is symmetrically enlarged and a bruit may be present due to increased vascularity. Besides exophthalmos eye signs include lid lag and, in more severe cases, defects in eye movement due to myopathy or conjunctival infection due to extreme proptosis.

452 Antithyroid drugs work either by preventing the uptake and concentration of iodide by the gland (for example, potassium perchlorate) or by inhibiting the oxidation of iodide and the binding of iodine to tyrosine (for example, carbimazole). Carbimazole is the most commonly used drug; once the patient has been rendered euthyroid a maintenance dose is continued for 1 to 2 years. Propranolol is used to counteract the cardiovascular effects of thyrotoxicosis and is particularly useful in the pre-operative preparation of a thyrotoxic patient.

453 Radioactive iodine is usually reserved for patients over the age of 40 because of the dangers of radiation to the gonads and to thyroid glands of growing children and women of child bearing age. It is particularly useful for recurrent thyrotoxicosis. It

is uniformly effective but there is a high incidence of eventual hypothyroidism.

454 In the United Kingdom, surgery is indicated when medical treatment fails to render the patient euthyroid; following relapse after carbimazole therapy; when the patient does not comply with medication; or if sensitivity reactions to carbimazole, such as agranulocytosis, develop. Surgery is the treatment of choice in toxic nodular goitre as this responds poorly to medical treatment. However, in North America, radioactive iodine I^{131} is preferred to surgery for most patients with thyrotoxicosis.

455 The patient is rendered euthyroid with carbimazole and propranolol. Lugol's iodine is given for a week pre-operatively to reduce the size and vascularity of the gland. The patient is admitted to hospital several days pre-operatively to check that she is euthyroid. Indirect laryngoscopy is performed to confirm normal pre-operative cord movement; serum calcium should also be checked. Two units of blood are cross-matched.

456 Most apparently solitary thyroid nodules are part of a nodular goitre, the remainder of which is not clinically detectable. A truly solitary nodule may be a cyst, a carcinoma or an adenoma — the latter may produce thyrotoxicosis. A thyroid scan will differentiate between functioning and non-functioning areas — so-called hot and cold nodules; cold nodules should be viewed with suspicion and further investigated by ultrasound and aspiration cytology or exploration, as 12% of these are malignant.

457 Surgery is performed for nodular goitre to treat or prevent compression of the trachea and oesophagus by the goitre itself or haemorrhage into it; to remove the unsightly lump; or if the nodular goitre has become toxic.

458 The specific complications of thyroidectomy are haemorrhage, vocal cord paralysis, hypocalcaemia and thyroid crisis. Haemorrhage in this region is particularly dangerous as it can cause suffocation. One or both cords may be paralysed due to recurrent laryngeal nerve damage; this causes stridor and hoarseness. Hypocalcaemia

follows accidental removal of the parathyroid glands and is manifested by tetany. Thyroid crisis, a very rare complication nowadays, is a very severe form of thyrotoxicosis, and only occurs if a toxic patient has been inadequately prepared pre-operatively.

459 Primary thyroid carcinomas may be papillary, follicular, anaplastic or occasionally medullary. Secondary tumours in the thyroid are very unusual.

460 The recurrent laryngeal nerve passes in a groove between the trachea and oesophagus and is intimately related to the inferior thyroid artery. It can be damaged during a thyroidectomy causing cord paralysis. By checking the position of the cords before surgery, one can be sure that there is no pre-operative damage to the cords or the recurrent laryngeal nerves.

461 Papillary carcinoma usually occurs under the age of 40, is often multifocal and metastasizes to regional lymph nodes. Follicular carcinoma tends to occur in older patients and blood-borne spread to lungs and bone is common. The prognosis with either tumour is fairly good, but particularly with papillary lesions, so long as recurrent disease is detected early and treated.

462 Papillary tumours are usually multifocal, with early spread to regional nodes. Many surgeons therefore argue that the operation of choice is total thyroidectomy and excision of involved nodes. Others point out that many of the abnormal areas identified histologically are of no clinical significance and they report very good results following lobectomy alone. As follicular carcinoma tends not to be multifocal, thyroid lobectomy may be adequate local treatment; however, total thyroidectomy has the advantage that it facilitates effective treatment of disseminated disease with radio-iodine postoperatively as this is then exclusively concentrated by metastatic tumour. In both cases, full thyroid replacement is given to reduce the TSH stimulation of any residual tumour.

463 There are three eponymous types of thyroiditis — Hashimoto's, de Quervain's and Riedel's. Hashi-

moto's disease is auto-immune and presents as hypothyroidism; de Quervain's thyroiditis is probably due to a viral infection and presents with pain and fever; in the very rare Riedel's thyroiditis there is dense fibrosis of the gland which may cause tracheal compression and laryngeal nerve palsy and is sometimes associated with retroperitoneal fibrosis. Acute suppurative thyroiditis is very rare.

464 Hashimoto's thyroiditis usually occurs in 30 to 50 year old females. Initially the gland is enlarged, smooth and may be slightly tender and at this stage the patient may be hyperthyroid. As the condition progresses the patient becomes hypothyroid and eventually the gland becomes fibrotic and impalpable. The diagnosis is usually confirmed by finding antithyroid antibodies though sometimes biopsy is required to clinch it. Treatment is usually confined to thyroid replacement therapy, though sometimes surgery is required for cosmetic reasons or to relieve pressure.

465 There are usually four parathyroid glands arranged in pairs behind the upper and lower poles of the thyroid lobes. The upper pair develops from the fourth pharyngeal pouch, while the lower pair develops from the third pouch and migrates caudally with the thymus, sometimes ending up in a retrosternal position. Identification at operation can be difficult unless they are enlarged but they have a characteristic yellowish-brown appearance. The glands selectively take up methylene blue and this can be given pre-operatively to aid identification.

466 Primary hyperparathyroidism is due to excess production of parathormone, usually by one or more parathyroid adenomata, though in about 10% of cases generalized parathyroid hyperplasia is the cause and rarely carcinoma. Secondary hyperparathyroidism may develop in chronic renal failure or intestinal malabsorption, both of which interfere with the normal dietary intake of calcium, leading to increased parathyroid activity. In tertiary hyperparathyroidism one or more glands, in a patient already suffering from secondary hyperparathyroidism, becomes adenomatous

and continues to produce increased amounts of parathormone.

467 Hyperparathyroidism may present as a chance finding on screening, due to the effects of hypercalcaemia or to the symptoms caused by abnormal bone metabolism. Symptomatic hypercalcaemia most commonly presents with nephrocalcinosis and renal calculi, but can also cause abdominal pain, muscle weakness and mental disturbance; in others peptic ulceration or pancreatitis develop. A raised serum calcium may be an incidental finding on biochemical screening. Other patients present with bone disease (osteitis fibrosa cystica, or Von Recklinghausen's disease of the bone) in which demineralization, the formation of bone cysts and 'brown tumours' (tumour-like masses of osteocytes) lead to pathological fractures.

468 Elevated serum calcium levels should be confirmed on several occasions and parathormone assayed. Typical radiographic features occur in the hands — subperiosteal bone resorption of the middle phalanges, tufting of the terminal phalanges and cyst formation. If on the basis of these investigations primary hyperparathyroidism is likely, the neck is explored to obtain confirmation of the diagnosis and to treat it.

469 Regular checking of serum calcium may pick up hypocalcaemia before it causes trouble. Hypocalcaemia may provoke spontaneous carpopedal spasm, while in others there will be Trousseau's sign (carpopedal spasm on occluding the brachial artery with a blood pressure cuff). Chvostek's sign (facial twitching on percussion of the facial nerve) or mental disturbance. Immediate treatment with calcium gluconate (10 ml 10% solution) followed with calciferol and oral calcium supplements is indicated.

470 Cushing's syndrome is caused by excessive circulating glucocorticoids. The commonest cause is medical treatment with steroids but spontaneous cases are usually due to bilateral adrenal hyperplasia, which may be secondary to a pituitary or bronchial ACTH-producing tumour. Adrenal adenoma or carcinoma are other possibilities.

471 The typical features are a moon face, greasy skin and acne, a fat trunk with thin limbs, hypertension and impotence or amenorrhoea. Abdominal striae are usually present and there may be marked osteoporosis. Diabetes is common.

472 Cushing's syndrome is due to a pituitary tumour in 66% of cases. It is usually treated by transsphenoidal hypophysectomy. Irradiation by external beam or yttrium-90 implantation is an alternative treatment. Where these fail then bilateral adrenalectomy can be performed.

473 Conn's syndrome is due to excess aldosterone production from the adrenal cortex, usually due to an adenoma. This produces sodium retention and potassium depletion leading to muscle weakness, cramps, polyuria, headaches and hypertension.

474 Adrenalectomy is the treatment of choice in patients with Cushing's or Conn's syndrome where hyperplasia or an adenoma of the adrenal cortex is the cause. This operation is now rarely used in the palliation of advanced breast cancer.

THE ARTERIES, VEINS AND LYMPHATICS

475 The two main symptoms are intermittent claudication and rest pain. Claudication strictly means limping, but by general usage the term intermittent claudication refers to a severe cramp-like pain, usually in the calf, precipitated by exercise and relieved by rest and indicates an inadequate blood supply to exercising muscles. Rest pain is felt in the toes and feet, is usually worse at night and relieved by hanging the foot out of bed. It implies there is severe peripheral ischaemia even under resting conditions and gangrene and amputation are inevitable unless arterial reconstruction can be performed.

476 About 70–80% of claudicants are unchanged or improved over a 5-year period and only 20% require surgery, with 10% needing amputation. In diabetics the risk is higher with 20–30% requiring amputation. There is, however, a 20% mortality in claudicants up to 12 years from the onset of claudication, mainly from myocardial infarction.

477 During sleep the blood pressure, pulse rate and cardiac output all fall, reducing peripheral perfusion below a critical level, producing pain which wakes the patient, who will often hang his leg out of bed to seek relief.

478 The patient may have Leriche's syndrome due to occlusion of the lower end of the abdominal aorta and iliac arteries. On clinical examination the femoral pulses will probably be absent.

479 The three areas most prone to atherosclerosis are in the arterial supply of the lower limb — the aorto-iliac segment, the femoral bifurcation and the superficial femoral artery, and the popliteal trifurcation and below. Aorto-iliac disease produces thigh and buttock claudication which, when associated with absent femoral pulses and impotence, constitutes Leriche's syndrome. Femoral disease produces calf claudication and the effects may be more severe than aorto-iliac disease as the limb is often totally dependent on femoral blood flow with little collateral supply at this level. Distal disease, that is atheromatous disease distal to the popliteal artery involving the small vessels of the popliteal trifurcation and beyond, is not usually amenable to surgical reconstruction.

480 The commonest conditions to be confused with intermittent claudication are sciatica and osteo-arthritis of the hip or knee. Sciatica often has a similar pain distribution to intermittent claudication and the associated paraesthesia in the foot can simulate rest pain. The pain of osteo-arthritis is often aggravated by exercise. Less commonly, a condition known as intermittent claudication of the cauda equina, due to bony narrowing of the spinal canal, produces pain and neurological signs on exercise.

481 Examination of the cardiovascular system should include assessment of the pulse and blood pressure, palpation of the carotid arteries and listening for bruits. Abdominal examination is important to look for an aneurysm. The lower legs and feet should be examined for their nutritional state, muscle wasting, pallor, cyanosis and areas of ischaemia and gangrene. The nails often lose their normal sheen and trophic ulcers may be

177

apparent over bony pressure points such as the metatarsal heads. Pallor and venous guttering may be provoked by elevation and cyanosis by hanging the leg down (Buerger's test). The temperature of the skin of the legs at various levels should be compared by simple palpation. Femoral, popliteal, posterior tibial and dorsalis pedis pulses should all be palpated and the presence of femoral bruits ascertained.

482 Femoral bruits are caused by turbulent flow in the femoral vessels and indicate significant atheromatous narrowing in the aorto-iliac segment.

483 The patient should be told to stop smoking, lose weight if necessary, avoid temperature extremes, take particular care of his feet to minimize trauma and the risk of infection, and to commence a programme of regular exercise which may improve the claudication distance. Finally, the patient should be reassured that his symptoms are likely to remain static or even improve if he adheres to this advice.

484 Claudication distance can be measured on a treadmill. Ankle systolic pressures can be measured using a pressure cuff and a Doppler probe. In normal people, the ankle pressure is unchanged or increased slightly after exercise but falls in obstructive arterial disease — the time to return to pre-exercise values is related to the adequacy of the collateral supply. Duplex Doppler scans, using simultaneous B mode ultrasound and Doppler measurements, give a clear picture of local architecture and flow as for example at the carotid bifurcation. Arterial flow can be measured by occlusion plethysmography, isotope clearance and electromagnetic flow measurement.

485 This is the ratio of the ankle systolic pressure to the brachial systolic pressure. Normally this is greater than 1.0. Claudicants usually have values less than 0.8 and values of less than 0.5 are associated with rest pain and indicate severe ischaemia.

486 Angiography should be reserved for patients in whom surgery is being contemplated, that is, patients with severe rest pain, gangrene, deteriorating claudication distance or in whom claudication is severely limiting their daily activities. The aim

of the investigation is to define the anatomy of the disease so as to determine the feasibility of surgery and the choice of procedure.

487 A transfemoral angiogram using the Seldinger technique, in which a catheter is inserted over a guide wire via the femoral artery into the aorta, is performed under local anaesthetic, but can be difficult if there is marked atheromatous disease in the femoral vessels. The images are enhanced by subtracting background images using a computer; this is referred to as 'digital subtraction'. Complications include subintimal dissection, extravasation of contrast, and haematoma formation in the retroperitoneum or in the groin with the risk of subsequent formation of a false aneurysm. Where both femoral pulses are absent a large volume of intravenous injection may be given, but this can precipitate heart failure in frail patients and gives inferior images to those obtained via an arterial puncture.

488 Atherosclerosis is a disease of the large elastic and muscular arteries. The earliest identifiable lesion is the fatty streak caused by subintimal lipid deposition. This progresses to the typical atheromatous plaque composed of cholesterol, phospholipids and triglycerides covered with a layer of collagen, while the internal elastic lamina becomes fragmented. The plaques are liable to ulceration and thrombosis on their exposed surfaces or haemorrhage into them. These processes may lead to stenosis or to weakening of the vessel wall causing aneurysm formation.

489 It is not clear whether atherosclerosis is primarily a disease of the vessels, the blood constituents or a combination of both. Cholesterol and phospholipids can cross the endothelial surface and excess lipid deposition occurs as a result of either a local increase in endothelial permeability or a decrease in the mechanisms which normally clear plasma-derived molecules from the vessel wall. Smooth muscle proliferation occurs in response to sub-endothelial injury and platelet adherence. The precise mechanisms which control these processes are unknown.

490 General advice regarding exercise, obesity and smoking should be given. Co-existing medical

conditions such as anaemia, polycythaemia, hypertension and diabetes all require treatment. There is little evidence to suggest that vasodilator drugs or those which alter blood viscosity are of any value. Acute ischaemia may be helped by infusions of thrombolytic drugs such as streptokinase or tissue plasminogen activator (TPA). These can be given systemically or infused via a cannula placed under radiological control at the site of occlusion.

491 Sympathectomy can be performed either surgically or chemically. A surgical sympathectomy consists of excising the L2–L4 lumbar sympathetic ganglia and the intervening sympathetic chain via an extraperitoneal approach. It is usually performed in patients unfit for major reconstructive surgery or in whom such procedures are technically impossible. A chemical sympathectomy is performed by direct phenol injection. The effect of sympathectomy is dilatation of skin vessels without improving muscle blood flow. Therefore it is useful in relieving rest pain and in promoting healing of ulcers but is of no value in the treatment of claudication. The benefit is temporary.

492 Atherosclerosis is commoner, occurs at a younger age and is more rapidly progressive in diabetics. In addition, the small vessels are often involved. Neuropathy causes painful paraesthesiae or loss of pain and temperature sensation. Motor neuropathy leads to small muscle atrophy and the development of clawed toes, which in turn leads to soft tissue damage by the shoe. Infection is difficult to eradicate because of impaired blood supply. There may also be abnormal arteriovenous shunting contributing to tissue hypoxia and increased platelet activation.

493 The most likely causes of an acutely ischaemic leg are acute thrombosis on pre-existing leg vessel atheroma or emboli (from the heart, from an aneurysm, or from an atheromatous plaque). Less common causes are trauma from a fracture or penetrating wound, an aortic dissection and vasospasm due to frostbite or ergot poisoning.

494 The patient's own long saphenous vein or a variety of foreign materials can be used for arterial

reconstruction. Autogenous saphenous vein is the best material for reconstruction below the inguinal ligament and can be used for coronary artery surgery, although better long-term coronary patency rates are achieved using the internal mammary artery. Teflon (PTFE, polytetrafluoro-ethylene) or Dacron grafts never completely endothelialize and so are thrombogenic, particularly at low flow rates and are therefore mostly used in aorto-iliac surgery. An alternative to saphenous vein is the glutaral-dehyde-treated umbilical vein graft. The Dacron graft may be woven or knitted in construction; the knitted variety requires pre-clotting of its wall but is easier to insert.

495 Angioplasty is a technique in which arteries are either dilated with a balloon or recanalized by passage of a laser through the lumen of the vessel. The technique is used in the coronary, iliac and superficial femoral arteries and is being investigated in the carotid arteries. Balloon angioplasty disrupts the atheromatous plaques as the balloon is inflated, whilst laser angioplasty destroys the atheroma by direct action. Whilst both techniques are minimally invasive the long-term patency rates have been disappointing. It is hoped that the use of expandable metal stents may improve the results.

496 This term refers to grafts which shunt blood, ignoring normal anatomy, to overcome ischaemia in patients in whom major aortic reconstruction is impossible, or contra-indicated due to inter-current disease or local sepsis. The commonest are the axillofemoral and the femoro-femoral crossover grafts; both are tunnelled subcutaneously. The axillofemoral graft is used in cases of bilateral aorto-iliac disease, whereas a femoro-femoral graft can only be used if a single iliac vessel is occluded.

497 The commonest sites for atheroma to develop are at its origin from the bifurcation of the common femoral artery and where it leaves the adductor canal through the hiatus in adductor magnus.

498 A trouser graft is a bifurcated graft made of PTFE or Dacron used for replacing the lower end of the abdominal aorta and its bifurcation. It is used to

treat occlusive disease of the abdominal aorta or aortic aneurysms where disease at the lower end is too extensive to allow anastomosis on to it with a tube graft.

499 A clinically significant reduction in flow is apparent only when there is a 70–80% stenosis although experimental work on pulsatile flow shows that much less marked stenosis has a measurable effect on flow dynamics.

500 The usual procedure is a femoro-popliteal bypass graft from the common femoral artery to the popliteal artery below the occlusion, or on occasion to the posterior tibial or peroneal artery if the popliteal is occluded. The best graft material is autogenous saphenous vein which may be removed and reversed or used 'in situ' after careful ligation of its branches and destruction of its valves. If this is unavailable or of poor quality then one of the newer graft materials such as Dardik bio-graft (glutaraldehyde-treated umbilical vein) or Goretex (polytetrafluoroethylene) should be used.

501 The important factors are graft material, distal run-off and smoking. Reconstructive surgery above the inguinal ligament with a Dacron graft has a patency of 75–80% at 5 years. Below the inguinal ligament where the flow is less, the 5-year patency is less than 50% in spite of the use of saphenous vein.

502 The indications are gangrene, ulceration, persistent infection and severe incapacitating rest pain in a limb in which revascularization is impossible. As a general principle the knee joint should be preserved to produce a better functional result; this can only be done if clinical ischaemia is confined to the distal lower leg and foot. Further, surgery should be more radical in the very sick patient who cannot withstand later revision, while it can be much more conservative in diabetics.

503 An aneurysm is an abnormal dilatation of an artery, usually due to atherosclerotic weakening of the arterial wall; these aneurysms can be fusiform, when the vessel is circumferentially dilated, or saccular, when there is an asymmetrical 'blow-out'. Aneurysms can also be

caused by infection (mycotic aneurysm), trauma and connective disease (e.g. Marfan's syndrome). The term is used loosely in the conditions known as false aneurysm and dissecting aneurysm.

504 A false aneurysm is a lesion in which the wall of the sac is formed not by the true constituents of the arterial wall but by organized fibrous tissue and haematoma, although the sac does communicate with the arterial lumen. It results from a contained arterial leak which may be due to penetrating trauma (knife wound, fracture, arteriography), blunt trauma, pathological rupture, or at the site of vascular anastomosis.

505 An aortic dissection is the result of a spontaneous tear in the aortic intima and inner part of the media, usually due to atheroma and hypertension. Blood then tracks between the inner and outer layers of the media forming a double-barrelled aorta. Untreated, rupture into the thorax, pericardium or abdomen usually occurs with a fatal result although occasionally spontaneous rupture back into the aortic lumen more distally decompresses the dissection.

506 An aortic dissection presents with severe pain in the chest, back or abdomen, which may mimic other conditions such as myocardial infarction or perforated peptic ulcer. As the dissection proceeds, the branches of the aorta may become progressively occluded causing ischaemia of the brain, spinal cord, gut, kidneys and lower limbs with the appropriate clinical syndromes.

507 Surgery is the treatment of choice in dissections involving the ascending aorta whereas those confined to the descending aorta are best managed conservatively, with controlled hypotension. The reason for the more aggressive approach in the ascending group is the likelihood of death from aortic valve failure, coronary artery occlusion or rupture into the pericardium if surgery is not carried out. On the other hand, surgery of the descending thoracic aorta carries a serious risk of spinal cord ischaemia and should therefore be avoided if possible; surgery may be required, however, if there is progressive widening of the aorta, indicating incipient rupture.

508 Abdominal aneurysms may be found incidentally on examination or when calcification of the wall is seen on X-ray. As they enlarge they may become symptomatic causing abdominal discomfort or, more frequently, back pain due to erosion of vertebral bodies. Pressure on surrounding organs may produce symptoms such as vena caval compression or ureteric obstruction. Rupture is often preceded by increasing pain but sudden rupture presents as an acute abdominal catastrophe or sudden death. Occasionally the aneurysm is found following massive bleeding into the gastrointestinal tract, or following embolism into the legs.

509 The extent and size of the aneurysm should be determined with ultrasound or CT scanning to define the upper limit in relation to the renal arteries. Surgery is indicated in most cases, unless the aneurysm is small (4–5.5 cm diameter) or the patient is unfit to withstand major surgery. At operation, the aorta is controlled above and below the aneurysm, the sac opened and a Dacron tube graft inserted. If the aneurysm extends to involve the iliac arteries, then a bifurcated graft is used.

510 Approximately 60–70% of larger aneurysms rupture within 2 years of being noticed and although the operative mortality of symptomless aneurysms is in the region of 10% this rises to 75% once they have ruptured. Thus if the patient is otherwise fit, surgery should be advised particularly if the aneurysm is more than 5.5 cm in diameter. For small aneurysms (4–5.5 cm diameter) treatment is more controversial and some surgeons prefer regular scanning and reserve operation for patients in whom the aneurysm is enlarging.

511 No, some aneurysms are not resectable. The minority of aneurysms that extend above the renal arteries may not be suitable for surgery as replacement of thoracic and abdominal aorta is a formidable undertaking. Inflammatory aneurysms, which are uncommon, provoke a marked reaction in the retroperitoneal tissues, so that surgery would be extremely hazardous. Various less radical procedures are being investigated, in

184

particular the use of endovascular prostheses introduced via peripheral vessels and expanded at the site of the aneurysm.

512 Iliac, common femoral, popliteal, subclavian, axillary, brachial and carotid arteries may all be sites of aneurysm formation. Occasionally multiple sites will be involved and this may have a familial incidence. A generalized dilatation of vessels with aneurysm formation at some sites may occur as a variation of atherosclerosis and is called arteriomegaly. John Hunter was the first surgeon to describe a treatment for peripheral aneurysms when, 200 years ago, he performed proximal ligation for popliteal aneurysm.

513 An embolus is a body, foreign to the blood stream, which is transported from one part of the vascular system to another. Pulmonary embolism is the commonest type, originating from thrombus formed in the veins of the lower limb. Also fairly common is arterial embolism from thrombus formed in the fibrillating left atrium or the recently infarcted left ventricle; less common cardiac sources are prosthetic valves and atrial myxoma. Arterial emboli can also arise from the material deposited within aneurysms and from platelet aggregations formed on atheromatous lesions in the carotids. Air embolus may enter the circulation via one of the large veins in the neck during surgery, fat embolism is a common sequel of major orthopaedic trauma, and tumour emboli may occur due to direct venous invasion, usually from renal tumours. Recently, therapeutic embolization using gelfoam or dura mater has been used to infarct tumours.

514 Emboli tend to lodge at arterial bifurcations, most frequently at the division of the common femoral artery. The effects depend on the size of the occluded vessel, the extent of the thrombosis which occurs secondary to the occlusion and, finally, the adequacy of the collateral circulation. Embolism to the leg presents with pain, coldness and pallor followed by sensory and motor deficit. If ischaemia is prolonged beyond 8 hours the leg may be lost. Embolism to the brain presents with stroke, to the retina with blindness, to the kidney with

pain and haematuria and to the mesenteric circulation with a sometimes confusing history of non-specific abdominal pain, with rapid general deterioration.

515 Heparin as a bolus injection of 10 000 units should be given immediately to limit the extent of secondary thrombosis. The operation is usually performed under local anaesthesia. The common femoral artery and its branches are exposed through a vertical groin incision and controlled proximally and distally. The common femoral is opened and a Fogarty balloon catheter passed proximally and distally until free flow is obtained. Angiography can be performed at the time of surgery and complemented by thrombolytic therapy. Postoperative anticoagulation reduces the risk of thrombosis.

516 Streptokinase and TPA (tissue plasminogen activator) are agents used to dissolve intra-arterial thrombus by stimulating thrombolysis. They can be used systemically as after myocardial infarction or locally as in the treatment of acute limb ischaemia. They may be introduced by the radiologist at arteriography or by the surgeon following, for example, Fogarty embolectomy.

517 Buerger's disease or thrombo-angiitis obliterans, is a condition of unknown aetiology which typically affects heavy smoking, young men aged 20 to 40. There is a progressive inflammatory process which causes damage to neurovascular bundles in the periphery of the limbs leading to gangrene of the fingers and toes. Treatment is far from successful and involves stopping smoking, sympathectomy and local amputations.

518 The surgeon will have been asked to perform a temporal artery biopsy. Temporal, or giant cell, arteritis may be complicated by the sudden onset of blindness, so if the diagnosis is suspected, it should be confirmed by temporal artery biopsy and steroids started immediately.

519 This is a syndrome in which the digital vessels, usually in the upper limb, go into spasm causing pallor, followed by a painful reactive hyperaemia in which the fingers become red and swollen and

subsequently blue. Occasionally symptoms are so severe as to produce ulceration or gangrene. This phenomenon is usually secondary to another condition affecting the arteries of the limb.

520   A variety of conditions have been found to produce Raynaud's phenomenon. These include atheroma in the main vessels of the arm, Buerger's disease, cervical rib, connective tissue disorders, trauma, ergot poisoning and occasionally as a result of working with vibrating tools.

521   Raynaud's disease is said to be present if the phenomenon occurs without a demonstrable underlying cause; this is most commonly seen in young women. Abnormalities of blood viscosity, plasma fibrinogen, immunoglobulins and digital artery patency have been detected in some cases. Treatment is initially aimed at protection of the affected part from cold; some patients require vasodilator drugs or sympathectomy. Recently, plasmapheresis has been found to relieve symptoms.

522   The classical mode of presentation of carotid atheroma is the transient ischaemic attack (TIA) which occurs as a result of platelet embolism from the ulcerated atheromatous plaque. A TIA may last from minutes to hours and is followed by a complete recovery, so the diagnosis is usually made on the history. Dysphasia, focal weakness, or focal sensory disturbance are characteristic, and visual disturbances, which range from blurring of vision to monocular blindness (amaurosis fugax), occur in about 20–30% of patients. Carotid atheroma as the underlying cause is strongly suggested by the detection of a carotid bruit. In about 30% of patients a complete stroke follows one or more TIAs, usually within 3 years. Sometimes a carotid bruit may be an incidental finding during a routine examination.

523   Five years after detection of the bruit, only 30% of patients will remain asymptomatic. Around 25% will have suffered transient ischaemic attacks (TIAs) and about 15% will have sustained a stroke; the remainder will have died from other causes (mainly related to other atherosclerotic disease).

187

524 The anatomy of the lesion can be demonstrated by duplex Doppler ultrasound, and if surgery is indicated arch aortography with selective catheterization of the carotid and vertebral arteries is performed.

525 Antiplatelet agents such as sulphinpyrazone and dipyridamole (Persantin), used alone, are probably ineffective in reducing the risk of stroke following TIAs (transient ischaemic attacks). Aspirin (300 mg/day) reduces the risk of major complications. Anticoagulants are of no value unless the source of emboli is the heart.

526 Patients who have had transient ischaemic attacks should have duplex Doppler studies performed on their carotid arteries. If these show a stenosis of >60% of the internal carotid artery then surgery should be advised to reduce the risk of subsequent stroke.

527 This is a condition in which exercise of the arm produces symptoms of dizziness, vertigo, giddiness and occasional blackout. It is caused by an occlusion or stenosis of the subclavian artery so that exercise of the arm provokes reversed flow down the vertebral vessels. A bruit is usually present in the root of the neck and the radial pulse on the affected side is weak or absent.

528 Acute mesenteric ischaemia, which usually results from an embolus lodging in the superior mesenteric artery, presents with increasing abdominal pain and with early development of shock. A recent myocardial infarct or the presence of atrial fibrillation may point to the diagnosis. The physical signs may be relatively undramatic in the early stages, but typically include generalized tenderness, mild guarding and absent bowel sounds. Unfortunately, the small bowel and proximal colon are often dead by the time a laparotomy is performed.

529 The barium enema shows the characteristic 'thumb-printing' appearance due to mucosal swelling in the affected segment. Sometimes this appearance can be seen on the plain X-ray if there is air in the lumen.

530   This is a rare condition characterized by post-prandial pain ('abdominal angina'), weight loss and steatorrhoea and is due to stenosis of the origins of the coeliac and mesenteric arteries.

531   A carotid body tumour, or chemodectoma, arises from chemoreceptor tissue between the internal and external carotid arteries and presents as a lump in the neck in middle age. These tumours are often slow growing but they may be malignant, the vagus and hypoglossal nerves may become involved and metastases occur in 20%.

532   Aetiological suggestions include failure to adapt to an upright posture, congenital weakness of the venous valves or vein wall, prolonged standing, pregnancy and a low residue diet. Extensive ileofemoral thrombosis causing venous obstruction and venous hypertension secondary to an arteriovenous fistula are rarer causes.

533   The patient is first examined lying down while skin pigmentation and ulceration are looked for. She is then examined standing (so that the veins fill) in order to record the extent and course of the varicosities arising from the long and short saphenous systems. The patient should then be asked to cough — a thrill in the groin indicates spheno-femoral incompetence. To determine the precise level of other incompetent communications between the deep and superficial systems, the patient is asked to lie down and a tourniquet is applied to the leg after the veins have been emptied by elevation. Any rapid filling of the superficial system below the tourniquet, after the patient has stood up, must then be via incompetent perforating veins. If surgery is contemplated it is important to check the patency of the deep veins. This is done by exercising the leg with the tourniquet in place; if the deep system is patent the superficial veins become less prominent as they decompress into the deep system (Perthes' test).

534   Injection is the easiest and cheapest method and avoids admission to hospital. The sclerosant is injected into the incompetent perforators and a compression bandage is applied for 6 weeks while they thrombose; during this period the patient

must walk several miles a day to prevent extension of thrombosis into the deep veins. Surgery on the other hand, involves several days' admission to hospital, tying and stripping of the appropriate veins, but only 2 weeks of bandaging. Although the early results of sclerotherapy are good there is a recurrence rate of between 65–90% after 6 years. Recurrence following surgery is about 15–20% at 6 years.

535 Stripping of varicose veins removes either the long saphenous or short saphenous vein. This is achieved by passing a stripper along the vein, tying it in place and pulling so as to avulse the vein. Avulsions remove the smaller tributaries. Small incisions are made over these, clips are applied to them and the veins are pulled out by sustained traction until they break.

536 Venous ulcers are caused by poor skin nutrition related to inadequate venous drainage. This happens after previous trauma or venous thrombosis in the post phlebitic limb. Less commonly they occur as a result of varicose veins.

537 Thrombophlebitis is inflammation and thrombosis in superficial veins. It is often seen at drip sites or varicosed veins. It is seen more rarely as a distant manifestation of carcinoma (Trousseau's sign). It is managed by non-steroidal anti-inflammatory drugs, strapping and mobilization of the affected limb.

538 Varicose eczema is inflammation of the skin just above the ankle caused by venous hypertension. It has also been called lipodermatosclerosis — a term which describes the underlying histological abnormality. Typical appearance comprises shiny atrophic pigmented skin which may become scaly and ultimately ulcerate.

BURNS

539 This is a convenient method of burn area assessment in which the body surface is divided into eleven areas, each of which constitutes about 9% of the body surface; these areas are the head, each arm, the back and front of each leg, and the front

and back of the trunk, each divided into top and bottom halves. In other words, the head and arms are 9% each, the legs 18% each, and the trunk 36%. The remaining 1% is conventionally ascribed to the male genitalia.

540 The rate of fluid loss from the burned surface is directly proportional to the area burnt, so that the assessment of the area involved is vital in working out fluid replacement. Depth of burn must be determined as those areas where the burn is full thickness will require skin grafting. Deep burns also lead to destruction of red blood cells, so that assessment of depth and area combined help determine the need for blood transfusion.

541 The initials ATLS stand for Advanced Trauma Life Support. This is an American-based system for management of an acutely injured patient. The system emphasizes the management of the Airway, Breathing and Circulation. The burnt patient may have multiple injuries and the management of the airway, if necessary by tracheostomy, must be the first priority.

542 Capillaries in the deeper layers of skin and subcutaneous tissue that have not been completely destroyed become widely dilated and of greatly increased capillary permeability; this leads to a disturbance of normal fluid exchange, resulting in a loss of circulating volume as exudate from the raw surface, and as oedema. Correcting this problem requires careful fluid replacement. If the burn is not too severe this can be achieved via the oral route, but in the more serious case intravenous replacement will be required. By about 48 hours post burn the excessive fluid loss ceases, so that fluid replacement (as opposed to normal maintenance) is necessary only during the acute phase.

543 There are three basic causes. First, during the acute phase dehydration and reflex renal vasoconstriction to compensate this can lead to acute renal failure. Second, in extensive deep burns, the release of tissue breakdown products and haemoglobin can cause acute tubular necrosis. Third, in the patient who has developed major infection, septicaemia can lead to renal failure.

544 15% of total body surface in adults, and 10% in children, who cope with burn shock less well than adults. With burns less than this size, extra oral fluids are usually enough to cope with the pathological fluid loss.

545 The badly burned patient is usually very frightened, in pain and in mortal danger. Immediate attempts should be made to reassure and calm him and treat his pain with strong analgesia. At the same time all clothes should be removed to allow assessment of the area of the burn, so that fluid replacement can be planned. A good IV line should be inserted, preferably by cut down into an arm vein. In burns over 25%, a urinary catheter should be inserted to help monitor fluid balance. Sepsis should be pre-empted by early dressing with antibacterial creams, such as Flamazine, or with clean sheets as a first aid measure. Anyone with a burn of more than 10% should be started on a 5-day course of penicillin.

546 The first step is to estimate the burn area using the rule of nines. Next it is important to remember that the rate of fluid loss, and hence replacement, is highest in the first 12 hours, thereafter decreasing until it stops, usually at about 36 hours. A useful formula can be used to plan fluid replacement based on this changing rate of loss; the formula is based on the 'ration' of fluid, one ration being given 4-hourly for the first 12 hours post burn, 6-hourly in the next 12, and one ration in the third 12 hours. The ration for a particular patient is worked out by multiplying the percentage area of the burn by the patient's weight in kilograms, divided by 2, and expressed as millilitres of fluid. This replacement fluid is usually given as plasma. The patient must be carefully monitored, and changes in the rate of infusion made if necessary. It is important to remember that the usual daily maintenance requirement of fluid, around 2 or 3 litres of water and electrolytes, must be given in addition to the replacement rations.

547 This depends on the area of full thickness burn, as this degree of injury involves destruction of blood cells at the time of the burn. Attempts must be

made to decide what proportion of a burn is full thickness; if more than 10% of the body has full thickness damage, blood transfusion is indicated, roughly at the rate of one unit per 10% body area deeply burned. This formula applies to adults — special formulae are required to decide on the right volume for children.

548   The appearance is usually helpful. Erythema or the presence of blisters suggest superficial damage, while brown or black leathery skin, or translucent skin through which thrombosed vessels are visible, are signs of full thickness damage. There is a group in-between which is more difficult to assess — in these the pinprick test is useful. A sterile pin or needle is driven firmly through the skin into the subcutaneous fat. Pain indicates survival of nerve endings and hence of viable skin cells, while the absence of pain suggests, though does not prove, that a burn is full thickness. There can, of course, be areas of full and partial thickness damage in the same patient.

549   Regular clinical assessment is vital to allow adjustment of the fluid replacement as required. This entails observing the patient's colour, degree of restlessness, blood pressure and pulse, hourly urine output, haematocrit, and, if progress is unsatisfactory, central venous pressure.

550   Grafts are required in the treatment of full thickness burns. They can help decrease fluid loss and perhaps prevent infection if applied in the acute phase, while in the longer term, they produce a much more satisfactory scar than would occur if the wound were left to epithelialize from the surviving skin around the burnt area.

551   It is normal to wait 14 to 21 days for the slough to separate and for healthy granulation to cover the recipient site. In some cases, however, early excision of the burn will provide a clean site to receive the graft. A partial thickness graft is taken from an unburned area, preferably from the thighs or lower legs, but the arms or trunk can be used if necessary; the instrument usually used is the Humby dermatome. The skin is spread, raw surface upwards, on tulle gras and then cut into suitable strips to apply to the recipient areas. If very

193

large areas are to be grafted, the skin can be made to go further by making multiple slits in it; the graft can then be stretched, producing a 'string net' appearance. In circumstances in which the area to be grafted is so large that the patient cannot provide enough autograft, cadaver or animal skin may be used.

552   Uncontrolled shock due to massive fluid loss, and uncontrolled septicaemia.

553   First, a major burn patient should be nursed in a clean dry atmosphere in a side room, away from the normal activity of the ward. Staff treating the patient should wear gowns and masks when entering the room, and a 'no touch' technique used. The burn itself can be treated either by the 'open' or 'closed' method. The time-honoured open method involves allowing a hard crust to form on the burn, which effectively acts as a barrier to the entry of infection. Alternatively, the burn can be dressed or, more commonly today, covered liberally and frequently with a cream antiseptic such as silver sulphadiazine. This method is certainly more useful in patients with more than one surface burned, or if the burn crosses a joint surface, movement of which would crack the traditional crust.

    Staphylococcus pyogenes and *Pseudomonas aeruginosa* are the most important organisms. *Pseudomonas* produces more pus which will destroy surviving skin and float off grafts — it can also lead to septicaemia. Bowel organisms also appear frequently, spreading to the burn from the anal region.

554   The treatment can be summarized with the phrase Stop, Drop, Roll. The patient must be prevented from running as this will fan the flames and dropped to the ground to protect the face and airways. The flames can then be extinguished by rolling the patient.

555   It may kill immediately by its cardiac effect. The area where the lightning struck will have an irregular branched area of burn which will usually be full thickness. The current passing through the patient to the ground may produce burning of muscles without damage to surface skin along the way, except at the site of exit, usually the feet.

Bones may be fractured due to violent muscle contractions.

556 There are few definite rules. Patients with large areas involved benefit particularly from the sterile environment provided in special units. Those with full thickness burns to the face or hands, or with full thickness burns of any part adding up to more than, say, 5% should ideally be transferred so that expert repairs can be performed. Other patients' site of management will depend on the interest in burns of the referring surgeon and on the availability in the area of a burns centre. Special units will always help with telephone advice, even if they do not take the patient.

557 Those who have been exposed directly to much flame or hot smoke may suffer burns to the air passages; this is a very serious, potentially lethal injury. Any patient at risk of having sustained such an injury must be monitored very carefully, both clinically and with blood gases. Antibiotics and vigorous physiotherapy should be used to try to prevent the development of pneumonia, and tracheostomy performed if respiratory function begins to deteriorate.

PAEDIATRIC SURGERY

558 Yes. The highest incidence of incarceration with subsequent risk of strangulation, and also damage to testicular blood supply, occurs within the first year.

559 Every attempt should be made to reduce the hernia by taxis. Safe sedation may be employed. Herniotomy should be undertaken 48 hours after reduction. Only if reduction fails should emergency surgery be undertaken.

560 Umbilical hernia occurs through a weak umbilical scar, usually as a result of infection. This type of hernia resolves spontaneously in more than 90% of cases; if it persists, with no signs of getting smaller, it should be repaired around the age of 3.

561 Gastroschisis and exomphalos or omphalocele. More than half of the babies with exomphalos will have an associated abnormality — cardiac, renal

and/or genetic. Associated abnormalities are rare with gastroschisis. In exomphalos the eviscerated abdominal contents are covered by a membrane whereas the viscera lie exposed in gastroschisis.

562 Drooling saliva or choking on feeding. This predisposes to aspiration pneumonia, as does the commonly associated tracheo-oesophageal fistula.

563 Vomiting, failure to thrive and repeated chest infections.

564 By endoscopy and 24-hour oesophageal pH study.

565 Duodenal or small bowel atresia account for about 40% of cases (about a third of babies with duodenal atresia have Down's syndrome). Hirschsprung's disease is the diagnosis in a further 25 to 30% while meconium ileus, mid-gut malrotation and volvulus account for 15%. Annular pancreas and internal hernia are rare causes. Neonatal intestinal obstruction occurs in about 1.25 per thousand births.

566 Bile stained vomiting, abdominal distension, delay or failure to pass meconium.

567 Phimosis and recurrent balanitis.

568 Imperforate anus is one of the commoner congenital anomalies and might otherwise be overlooked in the first few days. Its severity can vary between an anal stenosis, in which there is no more than a membrane between the anus and the hind-gut, to more severe forms in which there is a large gap, often with a fistula between the rectum and urethra or bladder.

569 Vomiting which is not bile stained in a previously healthy child between 3–6 weeks of age. Patient examination during a feed will reveal the characteristic upper abdominal tumour.

570 Ramstedt's operation; pyloromyotomy is performed for this condition. It consists of splitting the hypertrophied pyloric muscle until the mucosa is free to bulge out. Pre-operative rehydration is important. Vomiting may continue for 24 to 48 hours postoperatively.

571 Intermittent abdominal pain and shock, passage of bloody mucus from the anus and a sausage-shaped mass of similar dimension to and in the line of the large bowel.

572 Ultrasound will reveal the presence of intussusception in most cases. Definitive diagnosis is by contrast enema. These days air is preferred to barium. At least 70% of cases may be reduced and cured by pneumatic insufflation under X-ray control.

573 The most common causes are anal fissure and juvenile polyp. Fissure is caused by passing a hard stool and usually responds well to aperients and local lubricants. The juvenile polyp is a hamartoma, is usually single and is easily treated by diathermy snaring.

574 Conservatively. It is important to be certain that the foreign body is not inhaled and is not stuck in the oesophagus.

575 These are congenital urethral abnormalities. Hypospadias is the commonest congenital defect and occurs in 1 in 350 births. The external urethral orifice is situated on the undersurface of the penis or scrotum. In addition the prepuce is hooded and the penis has a ventral curvature due to fibrosis of the corpus spongiosum. Surgical treatment consists of straightening the penis by freeing the fibrotic corpora and a new urethra created using skin flaps from the penis. Epispadias is much rarer — the urethra opens on the dorsal surface of the glans or penile shaft. If severe it may be associated with ectopia vesicae.

576 A hydrocele is a collection of fluid within the tunica vaginalis and in infancy it is due to a persisting processus vaginalis. It may disappear overnight after the child has been sleeping. Spontaneous resolution usually occurs in the first year of life when the processus closes. If it persists it should be treated by surgical ligation of the processus.

577 95% of testes are in the scrotum at birth in full term boys. This figure rises to 98% by the first year of life. Maldescent is more common in

preterm children. Orchidopexy should be undertaken in the second year of life.

578   A retractile testis. Provided the testis can be manipulated into the scrotum natural descent may be anticipated.

579   The commonest malignant tumours in childhood are neuroblastoma (which arises from the adrenal medulla or sympathetic ganglia), nephroblastoma (otherwise known as Wilms' tumour) and medulloblastoma.

580   Excision if this can be done without mutilation. If this is not possible, biopsy should precede appropriate chemotherapy or radiotherapy prior to an attempt at a complete excision after tumour reduction.

THE GENITO-URINARY SYSTEM

General points

581   Renal pain due to pyelonephritis, hydronephrosis or a tumour can vary from a dull, poorly localized ache in the loin to a severe throbbing pain with associated renal tenderness. Ureteric colic produces a remittent excruciating pain which typically radiates from the loin to the groin and often into the testes. Cystitis is usually accompanied by a suprapubic ache and scalding on micturition. Strangury is a particularly severe form of pain felt along the urethra and associated with an urgent desire to micturate and is often caused by a bladder stone. Pain in the prostate from prostatitis is usually poorly localized and felt in the rectum or perineum.

582   There are many lesions throughout the urinary tract that can cause haematuria but the commonest by far is acute cystitis. Tumours, stones, trauma, infections and other inflammatory conditions can affect any part of the urinary system and cause bleeding. In addition haematuria may be due to a generalized bleeding tendency such as thrombocytopenia or anticoagulant overdose. Less common specific conditions which may present with haematuria are polycystic kidneys, renal infarction, Bilharzia and tuberculosis.

198

583 Initial haematuria, that is at the onset of micturition, usually originates from lesions in the urethra. Terminal haematuria is usually caused by abnormalities at the bladder neck or in the prostate. Total haematuria occurring throughout the stream gives little indication of the site of origin.

584 This should always arouse suspicion of an underlying renal anomaly such as hydronephrosis, tumour or polycystic kidney.

585 Lower urinary tract function is dependent on an intact autonomic and somatic nerve supply. Thus, occasional patients with neurological disease, such as multiple sclerosis, will present with urological symptoms, such as retention of urine, so lower limb and abdominal reflexes and assessment of anal sphincter tone should be performed in all patients.

586 100 000 organisms/ml of the same species of midstream urine indicates urinary tract infection. Infection should be suspected but is not proven by the presence of protein or blood on routine ward testing.

587 Sterile pyuria is a term used to indicate the presence of significant numbers of leukocytes in the urine in the absence of organisms on routine culture. Sterile pyuria, particularly in an acid urine, is highly suggestive of urinary tract tuberculosis. Other causes are bladder tumours, stones and treated infection.

588 Providing renal function is normal, fluids are restricted for several hours prior to the investigation. A control film is taken looking for urinary tract calcification. An IV injection of contrast is given and films are taken immediately and at 5, 10 and 25 minutes with tomograms of the kidneys; compression may be applied to the abdomen to enhance filling of the renal pelvis. Later films may be required if there is delayed excretion. When the bladder has been adequately filled, an after micturition film is taken to assess bladder emptying. The immediate films will demonstrate the position, size and shape of the kidneys and by 5 minutes contrast will have filled the collecting systems and renal pelvis. The later films show position, size and architecture of the ureters and bladder.

589 These can be broadly classified into metabolic and non-metabolic. Stones may result from hypercalciuria, either idiopathic or secondary to hypercalcaemia as a result of hyperparathyroidism or Vitamin D overdose. Less commonly, excess urinary excretion of uric acid, oxalates or cystine will cause stones. Non-metabolic causes include infection immobilization and persistently concentrated urine.

590 About 70% of stones are formed from calcium phosphate or calcium oxalate in various proportions. Calcium oxalate stones occur either as small smooth stones, irregular mulberry stones or sharp spiky jack stones. Phosphate stones are usually a combination of calcium phosphate and magnesium ammonium phosphate often forming the large staghorn calculi which develop in alkaline, infected urine. Uric acid and cystine stones account for less than 10% of the total and are usually hard and yellow.

591 Renal failure may be acute or chronic. Acute renal failure, indicated by sudden onset of oliguria, often progressing to anuria, may be due to prerenal, renal or postrenal causes. Prerenal causes include severe, prolonged hypotension or hypovolaemia due to burns, haemorrhage, septic shock or vomiting; obstruction to both kidneys is a postrenal cause. Chronic renal failure is progressive deterioration in function due either to intrinsic renal disease such as glomerulonephritis, or to prolonged obstruction.

592 There may be a history of long-standing prostatism or previous pelvic malignancy. Examination may reveal an enlarged prostate, a palpable bladder or a pelvic mass. A renal ultrasound is the most useful investigation as it will reveal evidence of hydronephrosis whereas an intravenous urogram is of limited value if the urea is markedly raised. There may be a rapid improvement in renal function following urethral or ureteric catheterization.

593 Pneumaturia is the passage of 'wind in the water'. This is virtually diagnostic of a vesicocolic fistula, due to either colonic diverticular disease or large bowel malignancy. Other causes include infection with gas forming organisms and following

cystoscopy when air is inevitably introduced into the bladder with irrigant fluid.

The kidney and ureter

594 On initial palpation the enlarged kidney is usually smooth while a notch may be felt on the inferior border of the spleen. On inspiration the spleen moves down, but the kidney may not. A renal mass can be made more obvious on abdominal palpation by pressure in the loin. Finally, on percussion the spleen is dull, while the kidney may seem resonant due to overlying bowel.

595 Blood urea is measured routinely but is not elevated until there is a 50% reduction in renal function. More sensitive measures of renal clearance and concentration include serum creatinine, creatinine clearance, urinary specific gravity and maximum urinary concentrating ability after fluid restriction. Individual renal function can be assessed using a renal isotope scan.

596 The kidney can be abnormal in its structure, position or blood supply. The commonest abnormality is partial or complete division of the kidney and its collecting system into two moieties. The lower poles of the kidneys may be fused to form a 'horseshoe kidney'. Polycystic disease is another congenital abnormality. Rarely, one kidney may be absent. If a kidney is abnormal in position it is usually located in the pelvis. The commonest vascular abnormality is an aberrant lower pole artery arising directly from the aorta.

597 Isotope renography using Technetium^{99m} (99 MTC) DTPA or MAG 3 can usually distinguish between an obstructed and a non-obstructed system. Using a gamma camera a delayed accumulation of isotope is seen, with a delay in drainage following administration of frusemide. In addition, GFR can be calculated and comparison of function between kidneys or the elements of a duplex system can be assessed.

598 It is important for two reasons: to demonstrate a functioning, intact kidney on the uninjured side and to obtain information about the injured kidney. An IVU may reveal unilateral non-function,

suggesting major damage to the blood supply or varying degrees of discontinuity or extravasation.

599 Surgery is indicated for continued bleeding, the development of a mass in the loin, or secondary infection. At most, 25% of patients with renal trauma require surgery and the aim of treatment is to preserve as much functioning renal tissue as possible.

600 Acute pyelonephritis presents with loin pain, fever and rigors, sometimes associated with dysuria, frequency and haematuria. The main physical finding is extreme loin tenderness. Infection is usually ascending rather than blood-borne and in over 50% of patients is associated with an obstructive lesion of the urinary tract. The urothelium of the renal pelvis becomes inflamed and haemorrhagic and there is progressive parenchymal involvement sometimes with the formation of abscesses in or around the kidney.

601 A JJ, or double pigtail, stent is a plastic or silastic tube for internal drainage of the urinary tract. It is inserted over a guide wire and because of the 'memory' incorporated into the plastic attains a J or pigtail configuration at both ends — the upper in the renal pelvis and the lower in the bladder, both of which help to prevent irrigation. It can be inserted in a retrograde or anterograde fashion or occasionally, at open operation. Side holes allow urine to drain along its lumen. It is used for temporary drainage after open surgery such as ureteric reimplantation or after stone manipulation and lithotripsy to prevent obstructions by stone fragments or to prevent urinary extravasation if there has been ureteric drainage at surgery or ureteroscopy. More prolonged stenting is used to relieve ureteric obstruction due to pelvic malignancy or retroperitoneal fibrosis.

602 Conventional surgery is required for less than 5% of all renal stones and should be used only when there is an associated renal abnormality such as a pelvi-ureteric junction obstruction or ureteric stricture which requires treatment at the same time. Staghorn calculi, where there is a large stone burden with many calyceal components, may need many sessions of lithotripsy or PCNL (percutaneous nephro-lithotomy) to achieve

stone clearance and a quicker result may be achieved with open surgery. Occasionally when stones are associated with a poorly functioning kidney in combination with sepsis and chronic inflammation, nephrectomy may be the best option.

603 Pyonephrosis is an abscess within the kidney, originating in the pelvicalyceal system, whereas a perinephric abscess is outside the renal capsule. Pyonephrosis results from acute obstruction to the ureter or pelvi-ureteric junction, with subsequent infection in the distended pelvicalyceal system, leading to rapid destruction of renal parenchyma. A perinephric abscess usually arises from an abscess within the renal cortex and only rarely as a result of septicaemia.

604 The original Dormier HM3 lithotripter introduced into clinical practice in 1985 generated a shock wave from an underwater discharge from an electrode placed in the first geometric focus of an ellipsoid. This focussed the shock waves onto a second focus, the area of highest energy and the position of the patient was adjusted within a water bath using biplanar fluoroscopy to focus the stone. Developments have occurred in imaging shock wave generation and shock wave physics so many patients can be treated without anaesthesia or analgesia by direct coupling contact lithotripsy. Other modifications include ultrasound imaging and shock wave generations by Piezoelectric or electromagnetic methods.

605 Percutaneous nephrolithotomy is a minimally invasive technique for removing stones from kidneys without making large incisions. Under general or spinal anaesthesia a needle is passed transparenchymally using ultrasound or fluoroscopic control, usually into a lower pole calyx. A guide wire is then passed down the needle into the collecting system and a track dilated to the required size by passing a series of dilators over the guide wire or by using a balloon dilatation system. A plastic sheath is then passed over the largest dilator to allow access for nephroscopes. Small stones can be removed intact whilst large stones require fragmentation with an electro-hydraulic or ultrasound probe. A nephrostomy tube is usually left in place for 24–48 hours to drain the kidney.

606 Uric acid and cystine stones are radiolucent and account for less than 10% of all urinary tract calculi.

607 Primary malignant renal tumours are of three main types — renal cell carcinoma, tumours of the pelvis and nephroblastoma. Renal cell carcinoma (hypernephroma) is the commonest renal tumour and arises from the tubules. Tumours of the pelvis arise from the urothelium and are usually papillary transitional cell tumours but occasionally may be squamous if metaplasia has taken place as a result of infection or calculi. Nephroblastoma (Wilms' tumour) is a mixed tumour of epithelial and connective tissue arising from nephrogenic tissue, and is one of the commoner malignant tumours of childhood. Benign tumours, such as lipomas or fibromas, are rare.

608 Patients with renal cell carcinoma most commonly present with unexplained painless haematuria. They may also present with abdominal pain and an unexplained abdominal mass. Less commonly they may present with polycythaemia, pyrexia of unknown origin, anaemia or with symptoms from secondary deposits.

609 Renal cell carcinoma is treated by radical nephrectomy, through a thoraco-abdominal incision if necessary, excising the perinephric fat as well as the kidney. Postoperative radiotherapy may be given if there is evidence of spread beyond the renal capsule or if local nodes are involved. Pre-operative embolization is sometimes used to reduce vascularity or occasionally as an alternative to surgery. Transitional cell carcinoma of the renal pelvis is treated by nephro-ureterectomy as the whole urothelium is assumed to be potentially malignant. Regular follow-up is required to check the bladder, and the kidney and ureter on the other side.

610 ABO blood group compatibility between donor and recipient is essential as accelerated rejection occurs with incompatible grafts. The role of the HLA antigens is less well defined. The chance of finding a pair of siblings with the same four HLA antigens in common is 1 in 4; in kidneys transplanted between siblings, 1-year graft survival is significantly better in HLA identical grafts (90%)

compared to non-identical grafts (70%). The results of parent-to-child grafting are similar to those in non-identical siblings.

611 Live, related donors with good HLA match are the ideal, producing about an 80% 1-year graft survival compared to 50% for kidneys from unrelated cadavers. Kidneys removed from cadavers often require preservation for several hours whilst the recipient is prepared, so that some are non-viable at the time of transplantation.

612 The most commonly used regime to prevent rejection used to be a combination of corticosteroids and azathioprine, with higher doses of steroids to treat episodes of rejection. Continuous steroid administration produces many problems and so cyclosporin A, either alone or with low doses of steroids, has become the principle drug for maintaining remission. However, it can itself produce renal failure and so the levels of the drug must be closely monitored. Antilymphocyte globulin and plasmapheresis are advocated by some but their use is controversial.

613 Urinary fistulae or obstruction may occur due to ischaemia of the lower end of the ureter. These can be avoided by routine use of a JJ stent. Early vascular complications are unusual but late renal artery stenosis may occur and present as hypertension and deteriorating renal function. It may be amenable to balloon angioplasty. Lymphoceles can accumulate and become symptomatic by causing ureteric obstruction. Diabetics are prone to cardiovascular complications. Rejection may be hyperacute, acute or chronic and anti-rejection drugs can all have complications. Azothiaprine can cause marrow depression and occasional hepatotoxicity and is associated with increased risk of late tumours developing. Cyclosporin can cause dose dependent nephrotoxicity but can also cause tremor and paraesthesia, hirsutism and gingival hypertrophy.

614 Part or all of the collecting system (renal pelvis and ureter) may be duplicated forming a duplex system. In complete duplication there are separate collecting systems draining the upper and lower poles of the kidney, with their ureters entering the bladder separately. The ureter draining the

upper part of the kidney always enters the bladder lower than that draining the lower pole, and may end at an ectopic site such as the bladder neck or urethra. In lesser degrees of this abnormality, the renal pelvis is duplicated, together with a varying proportion of the ureter, the separate systems joining to produce one ureteric opening into the bladder.

615 Bilateral hydronephrosis is usually due to conditions obstructing the lower urinary tract such as urethral stricture, benign prostatic enlargement and carcinoma of the prostate or bladder. Advanced carcinoma of cervix or uterine body may involve both ureters. Bilateral ureteric obstruction occurs in retroperitoneal fibrosis and rarely with abdominal aortic aneurysms.

616 The patient complains of episodes of severe loin pain, often provoked by a diuresis. An intravenous urogram should be performed following the intake of a large volume of fluid; typically this will show a grossly distended renal pelvis with a normal ureter. Renography will confirm obstruction. Surgical treatment consists of a pyeloplasty in which the pelvi-ureteric junction is reconstructed either by resection and re-anastomosis (Anderson-Hynes operation) or by rotating a flap of the excess tissue of the renal pelvis to widen the narrowed segment (Culp's operation).

617 Urine should be tested for blood and an emergency IVU performed to confirm the diagnosis. The patient is given pethidine and an antispasmodic. In most cases the calculus will be passed in the urine, which should be sieved in order to recover it, for analysis. Progress of the calculus may be followed with plain X-rays. Screening tests for underlying metabolic abnormality include serum calcium (to exclude hyperparathyroidism), 24-hour urinary calcium (to identify idiopathic hypercalciuria) and urinary cystine and uric acid.

618 Providing the stone can be visualized and focused, ESWL (extra-corporeal-shockwave-lithotripsy) could be used. Most stones will fragment better if they can be disimpacted by passing a retrograde catheter up to the stone and flushing it back into the kidney immediately prior to

lithotripsy — so-called 'push bang' technique. If ESWL is not available, then the stone could be flushed back and removed percutaneously — a 'push perc'. Alternatively, the stone could be flushed back into the kidney and a JJ stent inserted to prevent it slipping back into the ureter and ESWL planned as an elective procedure at a later date. Open surgery (5%) would only be indicated if the above techniques failed, particularly if associated with obstruction and sepsis.

619 Indications for surgery are complete obstruction; obstruction involving both or a single functioning kidney; the presence of infection; a stone judged too large to pass; repeated attacks of pain without progress of the stone; growth of the calculus; and association with an anatomical abnormality, such as a pelvi-ureteric junction obstruction.

620 This is a condition in which dense fibrosis occurs in the retroperitoneum, usually at the pelvic brim, encasing the ureters and obstructing them. The aetiology is unknown although methy-sergide, used in the treatment of migraine has been implicated; occasionally a malignant variety occurs in which retroperitoneal lymphatics become permeated with carcinoma from prostate, pancreas or breast.

621 The commonest cause is iatrogenic trauma during pelvic surgery. The upper ureter is occasionally injured by hyperextension injuries to the spine. The lower end of the ureter can be damaged by diathermy within the bladder or during Dormia basket extraction of a ureteric calculus.

622 Vesico-ureteric reflux is retrograde flow of urine from the bladder into the ureter during micturition. Reflux is relatively common in infants, but diminishes with age as growth of the bladder base tends to improve the competence of the mechanism at the vesico-ureteric junction. The diagnosis is made on a micturating cysto-urethrogram.

623 The aims of treatment are the prevention of recurrent infection; the reduction of reflux; and the minimizing of renal damage. Infections are treated promptly with appropriate antibiotics and long-term, low dose prophylactic antibiotics are

used to prevent recurrent infections. Effective bladder emptying should be accomplished by practising double or triple micturition. The degree of reflux is assessed by micturating cystography and progress monitored with 3-monthly urine cultures, yearly IVUs and renograms. Indications for ureteric reimplantation are failure to prevent recurrent infection; gross reflux; and progressive renal damage.

The bladder, prostate and urethra

624 Some patients may present with acute painful urinary retention. This may be preceded by obstruction symptoms such as hesitancy, a poor or discontinuous urinary flow, terminal dribbling and a sensation of incomplete bladder emptying or irritative symptoms due to secondary detrusor instability such as frequency, urgency and incontinence. Chronic retention may be more insidious in origin with gradual deterioration in health due to renal failure, or with nocturnal enuresis due to overflow incontinence.

625 The commonest cause is acute bacterial infection. In women this can occur without any obvious predisposing factor, while in men it is often a sequel to bladder outflow obstruction, its complications and treatment with a catheter. Sexually active women often complain of the symptoms of cystitis without demonstrable infection. Chronic cystitis may be due to tuberculosis, schistosomiasis or radiotherapy.

626 Interstitial cystitis is an auto-immune disease characterized by irritative voiding symptoms, the absence of objective evidence of other diseases that could cause these symptoms and typical cystopic appearances. The symptoms are typically of unremitting frequency and urgency with suprapubic or pelvic pain which is often temporarily relieved by voiding. Other chronic inflammatory conditions such as recurrent bacterial infections, tuberculosis, schistosomiasis and carcinoma all need active exclusion by appropriate investigations. Typically, the bladder exhibits petechial haemorrhages in the dome following distension under anaesthesia. Biopsies usually

show features of non-specific inflammation and there may be a predominance of mast cells in the bladder wall. Treatment is unsatisfactory. Approximately 30% of patients will get temporary or more prolonged symptomatic relief following hydrostatic balloon dilatations. Bladder instillations with DMSO (dimethyl sulphoxide) either alone or in combination with lignocaine or steroids may produce symptomatic improvement in some patients. More resistant cases may eventually require substitution cystoplasty or even urinary diversion.

627   As outflow resistance increases the detrusor muscle undergoes compensatory hypertrophy causing trabeculation, sacculation and later, the development of diverticula and ureteric reflux. The detrusor is unable fully to overcome outflow resistance so that there is premature closure of the bladder neck, leaving a residue of urine. Ultimately, the bladder may become a chronically distended atonic bag.

628   Exposure to the aromatic amines, benzidine, beta and alpha naphthylamine, has been found to increase the risk of developing bladder cancer thirty-fold. These substances are used in the chemical, rubber and cable industries; rat catchers used to use alpha naphthylurea in their poisons.

629   The usual presenting symptom is painless haematuria. Later frequency, dysuria and strangury develop and if the ureters become obstructed the patient may develop renal failure. Presentation due to spread outside the bladder is uncommon.

630   Transitional cell carcinoma accounts for 95% of cases. Squamous cell lesions may develop in areas of squamous metaplasia caused by stones or chronic infection or within a diverticulum. Adenocarcinoma, associated with urachal remnants or ectopia vesicae, is rare.

631   All patients with painless haematuria should be investigated with an IVU, cystoscopy and biopsy if appropriate. Urine cytology may be a useful screening test in groups at risk. Tumours are staged by depth of invasion:

Tis – in situ carcinoma
T1 – papillary tumour not extending beyond
lamina propria
T2 – invasion of superficial muscle
T3 – invasion of deep muscle or perivesical
tissues
T4 – invasion of adjoining organs.

Staging is based on the cystoscopic appearance and careful bimanual examination under anaesthesia. Biopsies must include muscle wall to allow the pathologist to assess the degree of invasion. More recently, ultrasound and CT scanning have helped in staging.

632 Depending on the extent of the lesion, bladder cancer may be treated by transurethral resection (TUR), radiotherapy, chemotherapy or cystectomy. Superficial papillary tumours, 80% of the total, are dealt with by TUR, followed by regular check cystoscopy. About half recur and are treated with diathermy or TUR; superficial recurrence beyond endoscopic control may be treated with intravesical chemotherapy. Tumours extending deeply into muscle or beyond are managed with various combinations of radical radiotherapy, chemotherapy, and partial or total cystectomy, depending on the extent of invasion.

633 An ileal conduit is an artificial bladder, made from a segment of ileum which has been isolated with its blood supply. The ureters are implanted at one end and a spout ileostomy fashioned at the other. The indications for this procedure are total cystectomy for malignancy or to bypass a severely malfunctioning bladder as may occur in spina bifida and other neurological problems.

634 Bladder diverticula usually result from the increased pressure due to outflow obstruction, and follow compensatory detrusor hypertrophy, trabeculation and sacculation. They cause incomplete bladder emptying, stasis, infection, calculus formation and sometimes squamous carcinoma after metaplasia has occurred.

635 Urinary incontinence is an involuntary act of micturition which occurs when the intravesical pressure exceeds urethral resistance; the patient is either unaware that it is happening or, if aware,

cannot control it. The term enuresis refers to incontinence, usually nocturnal, in children without detectable organic disease and represents a persistence of an infantile pattern of bladder activity.

636 In cases of incontinence, urodynamic studies help to distinguish between increased bladder pressure (due, for example, to uninhibited detrusor contractions — the so-called unstable bladder) and reduced sphincter resistance (due to sphincter damage or weakness). These studies find a particular use in the investigation of post prostatectomy incontinence, which may be found to be due to uninhibited detrusor contractions rather than a damaged urethral sphincter.

637 Careful clinical, radiographic and urodynamic assessments are important. Depending on the aetiology, treatment may include catheterization, external appliances, urethrotomy, prostatic resection or urinary diversion. Drugs such as anticholinergics may help uninhibited detrusor contractions and occasionally electrical implants may be used to maintain sphincteric action.

638 Acute urinary retention can occur without previous urinary symptoms or may be superimposed on a progressive history of increasing urinary difficulty; it is usually painful and the bladder is distended, tense and tender. Symptomatic relief is usually immediate once the obstruction has been relieved by catheterization. In chronic retention the detrusor muscle of the bladder has become large and atonic. Huge distension may occur and the patient is usually unaware of it. Dribbling micturition and overflow incontinence are common. In addition, due to the progressive effects of obstruction on the upper urinary tracts, there may be chronic renal failure.

639 Acute retention is usually due to outflow obstruction which may be caused by benign prostatic hypertrophy, carcinoma of the prostate, urethral stricture, clot retention, vesical stones or tumours around the bladder neck. Following surgery it may occur due to a combination of pain, anaesthesia and recumbency and in the absence of organic obstruction. Extrinsic compression from a loaded rectum and in women a gravid or retro-

verted uterus or pelvic tumour, may compress the bladder outlet. Neurological causes such as spina bifida, multiple sclerosis or spinal cord tumours should not be overlooked.

640   In a patient without previous urinary symptoms, adequate sedation and a warm bath may do the trick. Failing this the patient should be catheterized; often the catheter can be removed straight away and normal micturition will be re-established once the patient is mobile. If there are pre-existing urinary difficulties then an indwelling catheter should be left for several days. If retention recurs after removal of the catheter, a urologist should be consulted.

641   Bleeding may occur from veins in the wall of the bladder or from the kidney, due to reactive hyperaemia. Furthermore, a marked diuresis and natriuresis can follow, requiring intravenous replacement. Therefore, it is best to drain a chronically distended bladder slowly.

642   The risks of prolonged catheterization are urinary sepsis and urethral stricture. If the patient is in hospital there is the added risk that infection will be due to a resistant organism. To minimize these risks the softest, smallest catheter suitable for the purpose should be inserted under strictly aseptic conditions and a closed drainage system employed. For long-term use, silicone rubber catheters are less irritant.

643   Following catheterization, urine should be cultured and any infection treated. If there is evidence of renal impairment, fluid balance and anaemia should be corrected and catheter drainage continued until the patient is fit for surgery. Other investigations include an IVU and serum acid phosphatase to exclude prostatic carcinoma. A cystoscopy is always performed immediately prior to prostatectomy.

644   The size, shape and texture of the gland and the mobility of the overlying rectal wall can be assessed. The normal adult prostate is about the size of a chestnut and has discrete lateral margins and an easily palpable median groove. The normal gland has a texture resembling the tensed thenar eminence and the overlying rectal wall is

freely mobile. Hard nodules, loss of the borders and the median groove and fixity of the rectal wall strongly suggest carcinoma, while induration and tenderness are due to inflammatory changes.

645 Bladder outflow obstruction due to prostatic hypertrophy has both static and dynamic components. The static component is due to glandular enlargement and the dynamic due to smooth muscle activity around the bladder neck. Finasteride is a recently introduced 5-alpha reductase inhibitor which inhibits the conversion of testosterone to dihydrotestosterone within the prostate itself, thereby acting on the epithelial element of the prostate to produce shrinkage of the gland without jeopardizing potency. Some patients may experience up to a 30% reduction in prostate volume with improvement in symptoms and urinary flow rates. The smooth muscle in the prostate and bladder neck has adrenergic receptors, predominantly of type 1 and selective blockers may improve urinary flow rates by 30–50%. A variety of urethral stents made of gold or titanium have been developed, but are usually reserved for patients unfit for prosta-tectomy. Balloon dilatation of the prostate has also been used but the results are not very encouraging. Thermotherapy to the prostate delivered either transrectally, or transurethrally either as microwave or high frequency energy waves, can produce satisfactory symptomatic and objective improvement in selected cases.

646 Prostatitis is an inflammatory condition affecting the prostate. There are three types, acute bacterial, chronic bacterial and non-bacterial:

Acute bacterial prostatitis often presents with a sudden onset of high fever, rigors and dysuria and urinary frequency. There may be back, pelvic or perineal pain and the prostate is swollen, boggy and often exquisitely tender. Pus cells and organisms (usually Gram-negative) are found in the expressed prostatic secretions (EPS). Parenteral antibiotics are usually required and occasionally a prostatic abscess will require incision and drainage.

Chronic bacterial prostatitis consists of recurrent relapsing attacks similar to this. Prolonged courses of antibiotics such as doxycycline, may be needed.

Non-bacterial prostatitis may have very similar symptoms but bacteria are never isolated although occasional pus cells may be found. Treatment is more difficult.

647 Residual urine is likely to lead to recurrent episodes of bacterial infection.

648 Prostatectomy for benign prostatic hypertrophy is indicated when normal micturition cannot be established following acute retention; for progressive symptoms of outflow obstruction; when there is a significant amount of residual urine particularly if infected; for chronic retention with overflow; or when there are co-existent diverticula or bladder stones. Prostatectomy may also be indicated in cases of prostatic carcinoma.

649 Transurethral resection is the method of choice — this involves a piecemeal removal through an endoscope. The older suprapubic approach is not used very much these days. The aim of the prostatectomy is to remove the 'adenomatous' part of the prostate whilst leaving the rim of the normal compressed gland at the periphery.

650 Haemorrhage is the commonest implication. It may occur early (particularly if hypotensive anaesthesia has been used), or after 10 to 14 days, due to separation of slough from the prostatic bed. Haemorrhage may be further complicated by clot retention. Epididymitis occasionally develops, particularly if the urine was infected. Prostatic capsule or bladder can be perforated during transurethral resection and absorption of irrigant fluid into the circulation may follow. There is a small incidence of incontinence following prostatectomy.

651 Prostatic carcinoma most commonly presents with urinary symptoms indistinguishable from those of benign prostatic hypertrophy. Less common presentations are backache and paraplegia due to spinal metastases. Lymphatic obstruction can cause marked lower limb, penile and scrotal oedema. In some patients it may be an incidental finding on routine rectal examination or on histological examination of operative prostatic tissue.

652 The mainstay for diagnosis and tumour staging is with a digital rectal examination (DRE). Prostate Specific Antigen (PSA) is not useful as a screening test but levels greater than 10 mg/ml are suspicious but should be reviewed in the context of overall prostatic volume (PSA density), as measured by transrectal ultrasound (TRVS). Values greater than 20 mg/ml are common in the presence of metastatic disease. The extent of local tumour can be assessed more accurately by transrectal ultrasound combined with biopsy of characteristic hypoechoic areas. Capsular spread and seminal vesicle involvement are usually well seen. Bone metastases can be identified with radionuclide bone scanning. CT and MRI scanning may be useful in local tumour staging, but if a radical prostatectomy is contemplated laparoscopic pelvic lymph node dissection is required to gain accurate information concerning pelvic lymph nodes.

653 Patients found to have localized disease after careful staging, and with PSA levels below 20 mg/ml, can be treated in a variety of ways. For older patients with well differentiated small volume disease, there is a strong argument for no treatment — simply careful, watchful waiting. Only about 10% of patients in this group show evidence of progression over 7 years. More aggressive tumours can be treated with radical external beam radiotherapy or radical nerve sparing prostatectomy. Comparisons between these two latter approaches are difficult as the non-surgically treated group may be inaccurately staged as the status of pelvic lymph nodes is unknown. Radical nerve sparing prostatectomy is gaining increasing acceptance and the major complications of impotence and incontinence should be rare with attention to operative detail. Advanced disease is usually treated with endocrine manipulation.

654 Many prostate cancers are advanced at presentation either by spread beyond the capsule or because of lymphatic or bone involvement and are therefore incurable. However, about 75% of patients have tumours which are androgen-dependent. Stilboestrol is an effective agent but

has significant cardiovascular side effects and is now not often used. Bilateral subcapsular orchidectomy is easily performed but may have psychological sequelae; as 20–25% patients may have hormone resistant tumours, this should perhaps be reserved for patients who have been shown to respond to other hormone treatments. LHRH antagonists produce a medical castration by down-regulation of the hypothalamic-gonadal axis whilst anti-androgens such as Cyproterone acetate and Flutamide act by producing uptake of testosterone as well as some central activity. Controversy exists concerning the importance of adrenal androgens, but recent evidence indicates that total androgen blockade (with an LHRH analogue plus an androgen receptor blocker such as Flutamide) may produce better survival than an LHRH analogue or orchidectomy alone.

655 The commonest causes of urethral stricture are trauma and infection. Traumatic strictures may be due to perineal injury or pelvic fracture and usually affect the posterior urethra; sometimes they may be iatrogenic, due to catheters or instrumentation. Strictures due to gonococcal or chlamydial infection involve the penile urethra. Rarely, strictures may be congenital or malignant.

656 The urethra can be divided into penile, bulbar, membranous and prostatic parts. The bulbar urethra is vulnerable in direct perineal trauma and the membranous urethra in pelvic fractures.

657 Pelvic fractures are the cause of membranous urethral injuries, particularly when a central pubic fragment is displaced backwards. The prostate is fixed to the symphysis by the strong puboprostatic ligaments so that it moves with the bone fragment, tearing away from the membranous urethra. The patient is usually unable to pass urine and blood is apparent at the external meatus.

658 A urinary flow rate with a low peak rate and a prolonged voiding pattern is suggestive of obstruction but does not indicate the site or cause. An ultrasound examination of the urinary tract to assess the upper urinary tract and also the post-micturition residual volume is often combined with a flow rate. An ascending urethrogram and micturating cystogram confirm the diagnosis and

also define the length of the stricture, the degree of fibrosis and the presence of fistulae and abscess formation. The stricture can be visualized directly at urethroscopy which will allow inspection of the urothelium proximal and distal to the stricture. Depending on the site, treatment options are dilatation, urethrotomy and urethroplasty. Dilatation is rarely curative and often requires repetition. Patients can be taught self-catheterization with self-lubricating catheters (Clear Intermittent Self Catheterization — CISC) which will often prevent recurrence. Urethrotomy, which may be performed under direct visions or 'blindly' with a urethrotome, is more effective than dilatation. Urethroplasty, which should be curative, is usually reserved for failures of dilatations or urethrostomy, or far more complex strictures such as those associated with pelvic fractures.

The male genitalia

659 Testicular enlargement may be inflammatory, malignant or traumatic. Orchitis is painful and usually secondary to urinary infection or part of a viral illness. Tumours are typically painless. Trauma may rupture the testes and produce a traumatic haematocele.

660 Epididymo-orchitis is usually secondary to infection elsewhere in the urinary tract and is most commonly seen in men with prostatism and infected residual urine. Gonorrhoea, and sometimes *Chlamydia*, may be the cause in younger men. Tuberculosis should be suspected in chronic epididymitis.

661 The differential diagnosis is so difficult that, in the absence of unequivocal evidence of urinary tract infection, anyone under the age of 25 with spontaneous onset of acute testicular pain and swelling should be assumed to have torsion until proven otherwise by exploration.

662 Testicular torsion usually occurs in people in whom the axis of the testes is horizontal rather than oblique; this is associated with high attachment of the tunica vaginalis to the vas and gives rise to the term 'bell and clapper testes'. Sometimes there is a long 'mesentery' between the

testes and epididymis so that torsion can occur within a normal tunica.

663 Urgent operation is performed — the scrotum is opened, the diagnosis confirmed and the testis untwisted. If viable, the testis is fixed in position to prevent recurrence and the opposite testis is also fixed as the underlying abnormality is often bilateral. If the torsion has been present for many hours the testis may be non-viable and is better removed.

664 Almost all testicular tumours are primary. Seminomas account for 40% of cases, teratomas 30%, combined tumours about 15% and the rest are rarities. Teratomas are classified according to their degree of differentiation — teratoma differentiated, malignant teratoma intermediate, malignant teratoma undifferentiated and malignant teratoma trophoblastic.

665 Assessment of the scrotum is performed both by palpation and ultrasound examination. Clinical examination is performed to assess pelvic, para-aortic and supraclavicular nodes; gynaecomastia may occasionally be present. Pulmonary metastases are looked for on chest X-ray, while CT scanning may show abdominal or mediastinal lymph node involvement. Human chorionic gonadotrophin and alpha-fetoprotein are useful serum tumour markers.

666 This is performed via an inguinal approach in the belief that early control of the cord may prevent iatrogenic tumour dissemination. In addition, a scrotal approach risks contaminating a different lymphatic field.

667 Seminomas are radiosensitive and, following orchidectomy, radiotherapy to para-aortic and ipsilateral iliac nodes is given; subsequently mediastinal and supraclavicular nodes can be irradiated if involved. Five-year survival is 80–90%. Teratomas are less radiosensitive and require higher doses; disseminated tumours are untreated with intensive chemotherapy.

668 A hydrocele is a collection of fluid within the tunica vaginalis. In the first year of life it is thought to be due to inadequate lymphatic drain-

age and will usually settle without treatment. Children and toddlers with hydroceles usually have a patent processus vaginalis. In adults, hydroceles often occur without underlying testicular pathology but may be secondary to underlying disease such as tumour or infection. It is important to exclude an underlying cause by ultrasound or by cytological examination of the fluid and palpation of the testes after aspiration, especially if the fluid is bloody.

669 Idiopathic hydroceles can be treated by aspiration, though they often reaccumulate. Excision or plication of the sac is the definitive treatment. Some surgeons advocate injection of phenol solution after aspiration to prevent recurrence. In infants, communicating hydroceles are treated by ligation of the processus vaginalis. If secondary, treatment is directed to the underlying pathology.

670 Fluid from a hydrocele is a clear golden yellow, from an epididymal cyst clear and colourless, while the fluid from a spermatocele is milky due to the presence of sperm.

671 A varicocoele is present in approximately 20% of males with impaired fertility. A similar incidence can however be found in fertile men attending for a vasectomy. A significant varicocoele may be associated with ipsilateral testicular atrophy, slightly elevated TSH levels and reflux of blood down the testicular vein demonstrated by Doppler studies. Some patients may present because of a worry about a scrotal swelling and others may have persistent discomfort. Surgical ligation of the testicular vein via a scrotal, inguinal or high approach has largely been superseded by percutaneous embolization of the testicular vein or laparoscopic venous ligation.

672 First the response to intracavernosal injections of vasoactive substance should be assessed (PIPE — pharmacologically-induced penile erection). Papaverine is the most commonly used drug in variable dose. Patients with spinal injuries or neurogenic causes may be particularly responsive. Occasionally patients may find that after a successful diagnostic injection normal erectile activity returns. Others can learn the technique to

use at home once a predictable response has been established. If the response to Papaverine is inadequate, arterial insufficiency or a venous leakage may be suspected and require further evaluation, although the results of arterial reconstruction and venous ligation are disappointing. Vacuum devices are commercially available and all depends on the principle of placing a cylinder over the penis within which a vacuum is created which 'sucks' blood into the penis which is then held in place by a constricting band which is slipped off the cylinder to encircle the penis until intercourse is completed. If these measures fail or are unsatisfactory, penile implants are indicated.

673 An undescended testis is one in which descent has been arrested at some point along the normal path, while in maldescent the testis lies outside the normal path of descent. A retractile testis is one which, due to cremasteric contraction, appears undescended but can be coaxed down with the warm examining hand.

674 An incompletely descended testis may be located retroperitoneally in the abdomen or in the inguinal canal where it will usually be palpable. The maldescended testis usually lies in the superficial inguinal pouch, which is anterior to the external oblique aponeurosis, lateral to the external ring; rarer sites include the peritoneum, root of the penis and the femoral triangle.

675 70% of undescended testes are associated with indirect inguinal hernia. There is a higher risk of torsion and trauma. Fertility is at risk if the testis is still out of the scrotum after the age of 5 years because both the development of tubules and spermatogenesis are delayed. The chance of malignancy is increased thirty-five-fold and this risk is reduced but not abolished by orchidopexy.

676 As spontaneous descent does not occur after the age of 1, orchidopexy should be performed as soon as convenient after this and certainly by the age of 5, by which time histological changes can be seen in the testes. Orchidopexy involves locating the testis, mobilizing it by dividing all its attachments apart from the vas and its blood supply and then placing and retaining it within the scrotum, usually by fashioning a dartos pouch.

677 A careful history including past illnesses e.g. mumps, occupation history and drugs or chemical exposure should be elicited followed by a careful physical examination. Three seminal analyses should be performed at fortnightly intervals, each after 3 days' abstinence and delivered fresh to the laboratory. A hormone profile with particular emphasis on the TSH level is important. A high TSH level and a low sperm count or azoospermia associated with small testes usually indicates severe and irreversible testicular failure. Oligospermia or azoospermia in the presence of a normal TSH level may indicate an obstructive cause and testicular biopsy and vasography may be helpful. Occasionally an obstructive cause can be helped by an epididymo-vasostomy. Rare hormone causes such as hypogonadotrophic, hypopogonadism (Kallman's syndrome) may be found. Obvious abnormalities such as a varicocoele phimosis or urethral stricture should be dealt with. Antisperm antibodies may cause poor sperm motility and steroid therapy may help. Unfortunately, in many cases little can be offered, but careful counselling may help. Occasionally with newer techniques, even with low sperm counts actively motile sperm can be isolated and used for in vitro fertilization and GIFT.

678 Phimosis is narrowing of the orifice of the prepuce. It occurs predominantly in small boys, in whom it be congenital or acquired and old men. In small boys the normal prepuce is often not retractable until the age of 4 or 5, thus predisposing to balanitis which may cause phimosis. In adults, it is usually secondary to poor hygiene leading to balanitis. Paraphimosis occurs when a tight prepuce is drawn back over the glans and left, causing venous engorgement distal to the constriction, making simple reduction impossible.

679 Erectile dysfunction is an increasingly common clinical problem and although some cases may be psychogenic most patients probably have an organic cause. Vascular causes include atheroma affecting the aorto-iliac segments, following diabetes, arterial surgery or renal transplantations. Occasional patients can be shown to have premature leakage of blood into the draining venous system ('venous leakage'). *Blood disorders* such as leukaemia and sickle-cell disease may be

associated with erectile dysfunction as may neurological conditions such as diabetic peripheral neuro-pathy. *Surgical damage* to the pelvic nerves and spinal cord lesions and injury are also common causes. Occasionally *endocrine diseases* such as hypopituitarism, hypothyroidism or Cushing's disease may present with erectile dysfunction and many *drugs* particularly antihypertensives may be incriminated. Following a careful history and examination, routine urinalysis, a full blood count, urea and electrolytes and blood sugar should be requested. A hormone profile to include testosterone, sex hormone binding globulin and luteinizing hormone (LH) plus a check on thyroid function are indicated. In selected cases the following investigations may be needed — nocturnal penile tumescence (NPT) arteriography, cavernosography and cavernosometry, and assessment of response to intracorporeal vasoactive drugs.

680 The basic principle of the operation should be explained, outlining in general terms its irreversibility. As sperms are stored in the seminal vesicles distal to the site of vasectomy, two negative sperm counts at 12 and 16 weeks are required before the operation can be considered successful. During this period other methods of contraception must be used. Recanalization of the vas occurs infrequently, most commonly in the early postoperative period, but late failures, even after two negative sperm counts, can occur. Although the complications of scrotal haematoma, wound infection and epididymitis occur rarely, persistent pain is a problem in 1–2% of cases and is not always associated with sperm granuloma formation. There may be a long-term increase in risk of testicular and prostate cancer.

THE HEART, LUNGS AND THORACIC CONTENTS

681 To fracture a single rib usually requires a direct localized blow or a kick, or a fall against the edge of a table or wall. If a rib fracture follows minimal trauma or a coughing fit, we should suspect a pathological fracture, that is at a site where the rib is weak due to a secondary malignant deposit. If there is evidence of previous fracture on X-ray, we might suspect repetitive falls, possibly due to

alcohol. The commonest problem is pain and its effect on breathing and coughing. Less commonly the rib may penetrate the two layers of pleura and cause pneumothorax.

682   The term 'flail chest' is used when a group of ribs are fractured in two places so that there is an unsupported panel in the chest wall which moves inwards on inspiration (or paradoxically). This problem should be identified early in the assessment of the patient's breathing in the first minutes of evaluation of a trauma case. If the patient's breathing is inadequate at any stage, the appropriate management, in the context of multiple injuries, is endotracheal intubation and positive pressure ventilation.

683   Pneumothorax is a condition in which air has escaped into the space between the visceral and parietal pleura. There may be a direct communication between the pleural space and the atmosphere — an open pneumothorax — or the pneumothorax may be a closed one. Closed pneumothorax can be due to rib fractures, iatrogenic injury during subclavian venous cannulation, underlying lung disease or spontaneous rupture of a lung bulla.

684   In pneumothorax of any aetiology, if air continues to leak into the pleural space under pressure, it completely collapses the lung and further increase in pressure pushes the mediastinum across, impeding the function of the other lung and reducing venous return by pressing on the great veins. This may occur as a result of positive pressure ventilation forcing air out or because the collapsing alveoli will not allow air to return, acting as a one-way valve. The emergency management is to insert a large bore intravenous cannula between the ribs, to allow the pressurized air to escape. In a ventilated patient, the position is then under control. In a spontaneously breathing patient, the condition is much improved but complete management requires insertion of a chest drain by more experienced hands.

685   Pleurodesis is a procedure to achieve adhesion between the visceral and parietal pleura to prevent recurrence of pneumothorax or pleural effusion. It can be done by abrasion using a video

thoracoscope or with an irritant such as tetracycline through a tube. Pleurectomy is for the same purpose but involves stripping the parietal pleura either at an open operation or thoracoscopically. Decortication is an operation for empyema in which a thick fibrinous layer is taken off both the visceral and parietal pleura.

686   Surgical emphysema is air in the soft tissues which can be felt as crepitus. It tracks along tissue planes and is typically most marked around the neck, shoulders and the face. It implies leakage of air under some degree of pressure. It occurs with rupture of an air-containing viscus in communication with soft tissues. The commonest cause is traumatic pneumothorax where the breach in the parietal pleura caused by the same rib fracture permits air to enter the chest wall. It can also occur with spontaneous or traumatic rupture of a major airway or the oesophagus when the air tracks up from the mediastinum.

687   With an open chest wound air can be sucked freely into the pleural space on inspiration and the lung collapses away from the chest wall. Ventilation is therefore quite ineffective on that side and severely reduced in its efficiency on the other side. A non-porous dressing such as tulle gras should be applied over the wound after asking the patient to perform a Valsalva manoeuvre to expel at least some of the intrathoracic air. If the dressing is effective the patient is now at risk from tension pneumothorax so this should be looked for and can be relieved by removing and reapplying the dressing.

688   A standard chest X-ray is taken with the X-ray source behind the upright patient (postero-anterior or 'PA' film). In an emergency, it is taken from the front (i.e. an 'AP' film) with the patient supine; in these examinations free blood or air may be missed because they lie one in front of the other and no levels can be detected with the vertical beam. The mediastinum appears wider on an AP film than on a PA film. If the patient is well enough to move, it is best to use an erect film and obtain a standard PA view.

689 A patient with a tension pneumothorax should have this relieved and an intravenous cannula in an intercostal space will usually suffice until the drain and experienced hands can be organized. In the multiple injured patient with blood and/or air in the pleural space, a drain should be inserted. If the patient is very breathless this may have to be done before X-rays can be taken. The safest area is in the mid-axillary line, above the level of the nipple. This can be reached with the patient supine. The blunt dissection down to and through the pleura, is safer than the use of a sharp ended trocar which can severely injure the lung and any other structure in its path, making the patient worse rather than better.

690 It is possible that he has a tear of the aorta caused by sudden deceleration. The typical site is in the descending aorta just beyond the origin of the left subclavian artery; the tear can be temporarily contained by the aortic adventitia and the over-lying mediastinal pleura. An emergency antero-posterior chest X-ray can be misleading, but if an aortic tear seems at all likely, an urgent aortogram should be obtained, after referral to a thoracic unit.

691 Haemoptysis can be the presenting symptom with cancer, infection or infarction of the lung. The commonest tumour that presents with this symptom is bronchial carcinoma (70% present in this way) but it can occur with tumours, benign or malignant arising in the respiratory tract. It can be part of the picture of infective conditions such as tuberculosis, bronchiectasis, pneumonia or even bronchitis but the possible co-existence of carcinoma must be remembered. Infarction due to pulmonary embolus can present this way. The nature of the accompanying sputum and the other history may help in establishing a diagnosis but it is a serious symptom and should be investigated.

692 A patient with a pleural effusion is usually breathless, the severity depending on the size of the effusion and the respiratory reserve of the patient. The percussion note is dull over the effusion and the breath sounds are very diminished or absent. In the erect chest X-ray there is opacification

which extends upwards from the base in proportion to the volume of the fluid. The upper border appears to curve up laterally because the X-ray beam passes tangentially through a greater thickness of fluid. A fluid level is only seen if there is also a pneumothorax.

693 Pleural effusions occur with infections such as pneumonia and tuberculosis; malignancy, most commonly secondary from breast or ovary; heart failure; collagen diseases involving the pleura; and metabolic disease associated with reduced plasma oncotic pressure such as cirrhosis.

694 Patients with lung cancer usually present with new respiratory symptoms which include cough in 80%, haemoptysis in 70% and dyspnoea in 60%. Pain is a relatively late feature and is part of the presentation in 40%. Chance observation on chest X-ray is not infrequent but more commonly the patient has already had some symptoms leading to the request. Many patients present with manifestations of disseminated disease due to secondaries in bone, liver, brain or almost any site.

695 Cytological examination of sputum is a valuable non-invasive test, but if the tumour can be reached, direct biopsy through the fibre-optic or rigid bronchoscope is the best way to make a definitive diagnosis. Bronchial brushings may be sent for cytology and biopsies for histopathology. Peripheral tumours can be diagnosed by fine needle aspiration under X-ray control and the resulting specimen examined cytologically. For more extensive disease lymph node biopsies can be obtained by mediastinoscopy or direct exploration of the mediastinum.

696 Bronchial carcinoma spreads via lymphatics and in the blood. Lymphatic spread is first to the ipsilateral hilar nodes and then to the mediastinal nodes. Blood-borne spread is to the brain, bones, particularly ribs, vertebrae and proximal long bones, the liver and the adrenal glands. These may all be clinically undetectable at the time of presentation and should be deliberately sought by investigation. The results of staging will determine whether surgery might be beneficial and whether palliative radiotherapy is of value.

697 The differential diagnosis includes malignant and inflammatory diseases. Bronchial carcinoma is a common cause, in the appropriate age group, while symmetrical lymphadenopathy suggests lymphoma. Tuberculosis and sarcoid can both present in this way.

698 Myasthenia gravis and thymic tumours are indications for thymectomy. Myasthenic patients without a thymoma, in particular young women, are the most likely to get a good symptomatic result. Thymectomy is also indicated for thymoma which may be locally malignant or may result in a variety of syndromes including red cell aplasia.

699 An empyema is an abscess within the pleural space. It has thickened walls with fibrin deposited on parietal and visceral pleura and it contains pus. There is adherence of the lung to the chest wall over part of its surface. As with all abscesses the primary management is drainage which can usually be achieved by an intercostal drain and should be followed by systemic and local antibiotics. Traditionally an inch of a suitable rib is resected and open drainage is instigated. This old-fashioned management is inappropriate.

700 A bronchopleural fistula is a communication between the bronchus and the pleural space and is a life threatening complication of lung resection, in particular pneumonectomy. Typically it presents 1 to 3 weeks after the operation and results in air and infected material entering the pleural space, and pleural fluid sometimes suddenly and in large quantities, flooding the remaining lung. A lung abscess or cavitating carcinoma may rupture into the pleural space and produce the same effect.

701 The highest incidence of tuberculosis is in the immigrant communities, in particular from the Indian subcontinent. Those with reduced resistance due to malnutrition, alcoholism, steroid therapy, HIV infection or intercurrent disease are also more susceptible.

702 Thoracic vertebrae may collapse as a result of malignant invasion, infection or osteoporosis. Collapse due to malignancy is usually the result of a secondary deposit and a single vertebra is involved. Infection, most commonly due to tuber-

culosis, involves two adjacent vertebrae and there is a paravertebral abscess. Collapse results in wedging of the spine, squeezing out of infected material and may cause paraplegia. Osteoporotic vertebral collapse occurs in the elderly.

703   Immunosuppressed patients are at risk from otherwise unlikely organisms, in particular transplant patients and those having chemotherapy for malignant disease. *Aspergillus* can grow as an opportunistic saprophyte in old TB cavities. Primary infections are otherwise rare in Britain although in areas of the United States these diseases are endemic, particularly coccidioidomycosis in the South West and blastomycosis and histoplasmosis in the South East.

704   Those least able to protect their airways. This includes those with a reduced level of consciousness due to alcohol, drugs, head injury or anaesthesia. Children can inhale small toys or peanuts in the course of games. Laryngeal obstruction results in death by asphyxiation if not quickly relieved. Much more commonly the foreign body lodges more distally and, if not removed, the lung beyond it collapses and becomes infected and a lung abscess may form.

705   Mesothelioma is a tumour of the pleura. The usual cause is asbestos exposure. It originates on the parietal pleura and spreads to encase the lung and fix the chest wall. Pain and blood stained pleural effusion are common. Diagnosis may be difficult because the pathologist may require large biopsies to find the characteristic features. Surgery is futile, other than to make the diagnosis and sometimes to gain some palliation from pleural effusion by pleurodesis. Neither radiotherapy nor chemotherapy are very effective.

706   Any patient with a febrile illness and any cardiac abnormality should be suspected of having endocarditis. Any cardiac murmur or known structural abnormality of the heart should increase suspicion. The clinical presentation includes 'flu-like symptoms. Signs include splinter haemorrhages in the nails and splenomegaly. Blood cultures are essential to help make the diagnosis and guide treatment and should be taken

before antibiotics are started. Echocardiography is valuable in detecting vegetations in the heart and abnormal flow patterns due to structural abnormality causing or resulting from endocarditis. Surgery is important in the management of endocarditis and for prosthetic valve endocarditis is usually the only chance of recovery.

707 An aneurysm is an abnormal expansion of an artery with all three components of the arterial wall represented in the wall of the aneurysm sac. This distinguishes true aneurysm from 'false aneurysm' (in which there is a collection of blood outside the vessel, contained by connective tissue) and from 'dissection' (in which the normal arterial layers are split and the sac is formed by only the outer layers). The commonest aneurysms in the thoracic aorta in elderly people are atherosclerotic and in younger patients the ascending aorta becomes aneurysmal in Marfan's syndrome.

708 In aortic dissection there is a longitudinal separation of the endothelium and media from the outer layer of the wall of the aorta, typically involving half to two-thirds of its circumference. This may involve the whole aorta from the root to the bifurcation. It originates from an intimal tear which is most commonly in the ascending aorta. The lethal consequences include rupture into the pericardial sac causing tamponade or, if the dissection progresses retrogradely to the aortic root, occlusion of a coronary or acute aortic valve incompetence may result.

709 Careful control of the arterial pressure, observation for symptoms and signs of extension and aortography to diagnose involvement of the ascending aorta are important parts of the management of aortic dissections. Dissections confined to the descending aorta do as well with conservative treatment as with surgery. Involvement of the ascending aorta is an indication for early surgery.

710 The head and neck vessels may become occluded with aneurysms involving the arch causing ischaemic cerebral damage. The spinal cord receives part of its blood supply from the descending aorta and the adequacy of collaterals is unpre-

dictable. These complications may be a result of the pathology, investigation or surgical treatment and so should be looked for regularly during management.

711 Infection, heart failure and the development of pulmonary hypertension are possible but not inevitable consequences of the ductus remaining open. As with other congenital heart lesions the patient is at risk from infection which in this instance is an endarteritis of the pulmonary artery. The risk of heart failure depends on the size of the left to right shunt. Pulmonary hypertension with reversal of the shunt may result; this is known as Eisenmenger's syndrome and precludes surgical closure. The tendency of the duct to calcify is an additional and surgically important consequence.

712 The clinical findings are a reduction in volume and a delay in the femoral pulses compared with radials, and upper limb hypertension. There is a systolic murmur and sometimes a continuous hum, both heard best at the back. The narrowed segment of the aorta is just beyond the origin of the left subclavian and this obstruction causes the changes in the femoral pulses and the systolic murmur. Flow in collaterals is responsible for the hum and the proximal hypertension is due to a renal response to reduced pressure below the coarctation. On chest X-ray, the '3-sign' is typically seen due to prominence of the left subclavian above and a post stenotic dilatation below the coarctation. The ribs from the third downwards are irregularly notched along their lower borders, due to the enlargement of the intercostal arteries carrying blood from the internal mammary artery to the aorta below the coarctation.

713 The four features are pulmonary stenosis, a high ventricular septal defect, overriding of the aorta and right ventricular hypertrophy. NB. The surgery of congenital heart disease is beyond the reasonable scope of undergraduate teaching but it would be appropriate to know why, amongst children with holes in the atrial or ventricular septum (i.e. allowing right- and left-sided circulations to mix), some are cyanosed and some are not. A grasp of some basics like the reasons for left to right shunting across atrial septal defects might be expected of any doctor.

714 Mitral stenosis follows years after acute rheumatic fever and is due to fusion of the commissures. If that is the predominant problem, it can now be treated by balloon dilatation. This has largely replaced the surgical operation of closed mitral valvotomy. If the damage to the valve includes thickening of the cusps, thickening of the chordae and calcification, valvotomy or valve replacement on cardiopulmonary bypass is required.

715 Thrombo-embolic complications, endocarditis and valve failure may occur at any time after valve replacement. The mechanical valves are more prone to thrombus formation which may obstruct the valve mechanism or be thrown off as emboli, so all patients must be anticoagulated. Endocarditis occurs with tissue and mechanical valves, so all dental procedures should be preceded by antibiotic prophylaxis. Valve failure tends to be slow but inevitable with tissue valves and is less common but sudden and disastrous with mechanical valves.

716 The history may include syncopal attacks, angina, breathlessness on exertion and fatigue, but many patients are asymptomatic. The pulse is slow-rising and there is an ejection systolic murmur heard best at the base which radiates into the neck.

717 Coronary artery bypass grafting is indicated for the symptomatic relief of angina; it also improves the prognosis in certain categories of coronary artery disease. Patients with angina not readily controlled by medical treatment and severe enough to interfere with reasonable life style, should be considered for surgery, because symptomatic relief can be obtained in about 90%. A strongly positive exercise ECG, whatever the degree of angina, is an indication for angiography with a view to surgery.

718 Prognosis is improved by surgery in left main stem coronary artery stenosis from about 50% to about 85% 5-year survival and in three-vessel coronary artery disease from about 80% to about 95% 5-year survival. Patients with impaired left ventricular function also have an improved prognosis with surgery. In all but the benign forms of the disease where prognosis is good in any case, revascularization improves the chances of survival.

719 Angina pectoris means a choking sensation in the chest, from the Latin 'angere' to choke, and is the way patients frequently describe their symptom. Ludwig's angina is cellulitis of the floor of the mouth. In Vincent's angina a pseudomembrane forms on the pharynx and tonsils and two organisms (the spirochaete, *Borrelia vincenti* and a fusiform bacillus) are typically found.

720 Acute mitral regurgitation due to papillary muscle infarction and acute ventricular septal defect due to rupture of a septal infarct can both be surgically corrected. These operations have a high mortality and are only performed because the patient's outlook may be hopeless without surgery.

721 a) The overall mortality in the UK was under 3% during the 1980s. This figure is dependent on case mix and with more elderly patients (over 70) and more emergency cases, higher figures were reported in the 1990s, particularly from the United States.
   b) About 80% of patients can exercise without angina or anti-anginal medication at a year.
   c) Typical cases have a 90% probability of survival at 5 years but again this is dependent on the case mix and in particular age and the state of the left ventricle prior to surgery.

NEUROSURGERY

722 Yes. Intracranial tumours often present with late onset epilepsy. In this age group ischaemia and tumours are the commonest causes. Normal clinical examination and skull X-ray do not exclude a tumour and further investigation is essential to ensure that a remediable pathology is not present.

723 Severe headaches and neck stiffness suggest meningism resulting from either subarachnoid blood or infection. The mode of onset of the patient's symptoms is important in determining the cause. Subarachnoid haemorrhage occurs instantly, whereas meningitis is of more gradual onset. Subarachnoid haemorrhage may cause a transient loss of consciousness. History of prodromal illness may precede a viral meningitis.

If the infection is bacterial the patient may have symptoms of a source such as ear or sinus infection.

724 Difficulty in walking and micturition suggest a spinal lesion. In this age group, metastatic extradural cord compression is the most likely cause, usually from lung, prostate or kidney. In the female, breast carcinoma is the most common primary site.

725 Vertebral tenderness, a sensory loss corresponding to the site of the lesion and paraparesis progressing to paraplegia support a diagnosis of cord compression. A large bladder and a lax sphincter indicate concomitant autonomic dysfunction.

726 Yes. The presence of a skull fracture in a conscious patient increases the risk of an intracranial haematoma 400 times. Hospital admission should allow earlier detection of a traumatic haematoma, thus reducing the chance of secondary brain damage, that is, brain damage occurring secondarily to damage at impact.

727 The occurrence of a period of loss of consciousness and the duration of post-traumatic amnesia both indicate a degree of neural damage and reflect the severity of the brain injury. A history of assault with an instrument such as a hammer should raise suspicion of a serious injury, even if there has not been an episode of unconsciousness or amnesia.

728 Conscious level and pupil reaction to light are the most important features to assess in a head-injured patient. Evidence of limb weakness is also relevant. A single assessment is of limited value. Repeated assessments over a few hours on the other hand are valuable in demonstrating the trend in the patient's condition.

729 The Glasgow Coma scale is an objective and numeric scale for assessing the level of consciousness which was developed in Glasgow. The patient's speech, movement and eye opening are assessed after maximally stimulating the patient to gain a response. Verbal responses are scored as 5 for orientated speech, 4 for confused speech, 3

for words, 2 for sounds and 1 for no speech. Motor responses are scored as 6 for movement to command, 5 for localizing to pain, 4 for withdrawing to pain, 3 for flexing to pain, 2 for extending to pain, 1 for no movement. Eye opening is scored as 4 for spontaneous eye opening, 3 for opening to speech, 2 for opening to pain and 1 for no eye opening. Patients with a Glasgow Coma scale of 8 or less are in coma. Any deterioration in the coma scale following admission after a head injury may reflect an intracranial bleed and is therefore taken very seriously.

730   Pupil dilatation and failure to react to light suggest a third nerve palsy and are useful localizing signs as they always occur on the side of the expanding lesion. There is midline shift initially, followed by herniation of the medial edge of the temporal lobe through the tentorial hiatus. This herniation compresses not only the third nerve but also the mid-brain. Local damage to the eye may also result in a fixed dilated pupil.

731   Limb weakness is detected by observing the response of the limbs to painful stimuli. Any inequality in the response on each side indicates a weakness on the side of the poorer response. Thus, localization of the left arm to pain and flexion of the right arm indicates a right-sided weakness. Alternatively, flexion in the right arm and extension in the left indicates a weakness of the left side.

732   A skull X-ray is the first line investigation, but a CT scan is necessary to indicate the exact site, nature and size of an intracranial haematoma and to detect the presence of cerebral contusions.

733   The most commonly found lesion is a mixture of subdural and intracerebral haematoma where the latter has burst out onto the cortical surface of the frontal or temporal lobes i.e. a 'burst' lobe (35%). Approximately 20% of intracranial haematomas are pure subdurals and a further 20% discrete intracerebral haematomas. Extradural haematomas occur in about 15% of cases, the remainder being made up of mixed extradural and intradural lesions.

734 A fracture running across the line of the middle meningeal artery may tear this vessel and cause an extradural haemorrhage. Less commonly, extradural bleeding can result from fractures crossing the sagittal or transverse sinus.

735 Shearing damage to the white matter due to movement of the brain within the skull on deceleration, is a common contributory cause of coma in patients without intracranial haematoma. This may range from a mild injury causing transient loss of consciousness to a severe and fatal injury. Other factors include diffuse hypoxic damage, or tentorial and tonsillar herniation from diffuse cerebral swelling. Cortical contusions or lacerations, the common precursors of intradural bleeding, do not in themselves contribute to depression of conscious level.

736 Space-occupying traumatic haematomas require urgent evacuation through a craniotomy (a large bone flap). In exceptional circumstances, where speed is essential, burr hole decompression of an extradural haematoma may halt a rapid deterioration in conscious level, but in general, burr hole exploration outside a neurosurgical unit is not advised.

737 Chronic subdural haematoma occurs usually in infancy or in the elderly tending to cause a gradual deterioration in conscious level often with a fluctuating course, although focal signs may also occur. Chronic subdural haematomas may not present until several months after injury and in some patients no history of head injury is obtained.

738 After approximately 14 days subdural collections liquefy and are easily evacuated through burr holes. A subdural drain may be left in place. In a proportion of patients re-collection occurs and re-evacuation is required. Subdural peritoneal shunting or craniotomy are rarely necessary.

739 Yes. In this situation mere suture of the laceration would produce considerable risk of meningitis or cerebral abscess formation. The wound must be débrided, the depressed bone fragments elevated

and either removed or cleaned thoroughly and returned to place. The presence of a dural tear increases the risk of post-traumatic epilepsy.

740 A rise in intracranial pressure causes headache, usually worse in the mornings and aggravated by coughing or stooping. Vomiting may occur, often without warning. Examination of the optic fundus may reveal papilloedema. Since tumour expansion is slow, considerable compensation is possible, but eventually the patient's conscious level will deteriorate.

741 If raised intracranial pressure is suspected, lumbar puncture must **not** be performed in view of the risk of precipitating tentorial or tonsillar herniation in the presence of a mass lesion.

742 Preliminary investigation of an intracranial tumour must include a chest X-ray to exclude a lung primary. Skull X-ray may show pineal shift, evidence of raised pressure (erosion of the posterior), bony erosion or calcification, but either a CT scan or an MRI will be necessary to demonstrate the exact lesion site. Intravenous contrast may give more information by showing areas of blood–brain barrier breakdown or regions of high vascularity. Angiography is sometimes of value in showing abnormal tumour circulation and in demonstrating the exact relationship or involvement of blood vessels.

743 MRI is more sensitive to tissue changes than CT and can demonstrate any plane without the need for image reconstruction (which results in loss of image quality). These considerable advantages are slightly offset by the failure of MRI to demonstrate bone directly. In addition it cannot be used in patients with a pacemaker or ferromagnetic implant and in some a general anaesthetic is required to overcome claustrophobia.

744 In adults the commonest intracranial tumour is metastatic. Of the primary cerebral tumours, astrocytoma occurs most frequently, usually the poorly differentiated anaplastic type. In children, supratentorial tumours are rare. The commonest tumour is the cerebellar medulloblastoma.

745 In an HIV patient, toxoplasmosis or lymphoma are the most likely causes of intracerebral mass lesions. Bacterial or fungal abscesses or Kaposi's sarcoma are other possibilities. Invasive operative procedures are avoided in the first instance. A trial of pyrimethamine and sulphadiazine are given for toxoplasmosis and the effects monitored with CT. A failure to respond indicates the need for biopsy.

746 Yes, but this depends on the site of origin. A 'complete' removal must include the point of dural attachment. This is seldom possible when the meningioma arises from the skull base, the transverse sinus or the posterior two-thirds of the sagittal sinus. Incomplete removal greatly increases the chance of recurrence.

747 Acoustic neuromas present with a progressive deafness. Patients may also experience transient bouts of vertigo and tinnitus but these are seldom prominent features. With further growth cerebellar signs develop followed by adequate compression and hydrocephalus. Other cranial nerve palsies (especially the 5th nerve) may occur, but the 7th cranial nerve is remarkably resilient to damage despite its close relationship to the tumour.

748 Immunoassay techniques permit a classification based on the hormone type secreted — prolactinoma, GH secreting tumour and ACTH secreting tumour. (TSH and FSH/LH secreting tumours are extremely rare.) This supersedes the old classification of pituitary tumours, based on histological staining characteristics — acidophil, basophil and chromophobe adenoma.

749 Suprasellar extension of a pituitary adenoma causes compression of the optic chiasma, producing a superior bitemporal quadrantanopia initially, progressing to a bitemporal hemianopia. Less often extension into the cavernous sinus causes III–VI cranial nerve palsies.

750 The standard approach is from below via either a transphenoidal or transethmoidal route. These carry a low risk. Some tumours with large lateral

or anterior suprasellar extension require a sub-frontal approach to permit adequate exposure and tumour removal.

751 Not if CT scanning is available — this is the preferred method of diagnosing subarachnoid haemorrhage. If this is not immediately available, then lumbar puncture is still a useful alternative, particularly if there is some doubt about the clinical history, **provided** that conscious level is not impaired and that neither papilloedema nor focal signs are present. If the CT scan is negative, the presence of blood stained cerebrospinal fluid (CSF) with a xantho-chromic supernatant confirms subarachnoid haemorrhage.

752 Arteriovenous malformation, tumour, anticoagulant treatment or a bleeding diathesis may cause subarachnoid haemorrhage. However, in approximately 30% of patients even after four-vessel angiography the cause will not have been discovered.

753 Expansion or rupture of an aneurysm arising from the origin of the posterior communicating artery (or occasionally from the basilar bifurcation) may cause a third nerve palsy due to direct pressure.

754 A CT scan usually confirms the presence of subarachnoid blood and by demonstrating a focal collection may suggest the site of an aneurysm. This is especially useful if multiple aneurysms are present. Irrespective of the CT scan findings, angiography is still required to determine and delineate the exact nature of the lesion.

755 About 60% of patients survive the initial aneurysm rupture but subsequent mortality risks are high. The aneurysm may rebleed, causing death in two out of three patients. The rebleed risk diminishes with time but never disappears. Breakdown products of blood in contact with the intracranial vessels cause vasospasm in 50% of patients and many develop clinical evidence of cerebral ischaemia. Finally the presence of blood in the CSF may block its normal route of absorption at the arachnoid villi causing a communicating hydrocephalus.

756   In the first 6 months approximately 40% of survivors of the initial aneurysm rupture rebleed; of these two-thirds die. Beyond the first 6 months after aneurysm rupture, the risk of rebleeding is 3.5% per year; again two-thirds of the patients rebleeding die. Thus the risk of death from rebleeding after the first 6 months is 25% over a 10-year period.

757   Clipping of the aneurysm neck at operation is the only certain way of preventing rebleeding. Inducing thrombosis within the aneurysm sac by introducing fine platinum coils via the intravascular route provides an alternative method, but results await full evaluation. Antifibrinolytic drugs reduce rebleeding by preventing clot resorption around the aneurysm fundus but their benefit is offset by an increased risk of cerebral ischaemia, so they should not be used. Reactive hypertension commonly occurs after subarachnoid haemorrhage. Any attempt at reducing blood pressure using antihypertensive drugs although reducing rebleeding, also risks cerebral ischaemia.

758   Arteriovenous malformations usually present with subarachnoid haemorrhage but many present with epilepsy. In a few, focal signs or signs of raised intracranial pressure predominate.

759   Straight spinal X-rays in a patient with metastatic cord compression may show erosion of the pedicle, collapse or erosion of the vertebral body or a paravertebral mass. These features should correspond with the patient's sensory level. If not, multiple lesions must be considered.

760   Tumours, infective and degenerative lesions are the main benign causes of cord compression. Tumours include neurofibroma, meningioma, lipoma and dermoid/epidermoid cysts. Infective lesions may be acute staphylococcal or chronic tuberculous. Cord compression from osteo-arthritic degeneration usually occurs in the cervical spine. Rarely, acute disc protrusion and angiomatous malformation may present in this manner.

761   A lateral disc protrusion at L5/S1 level usually compresses the S1 nerve root. This causes leg

pain radiating down to the lateral aspect of the foot or sole. The pain is typically aggravated by coughing or straining. Signs of S1 root compression include weakness of the plantar flexors and invertors of the foot, impaired sensation over the lateral border of the foot and a diminished or absent ankle jerk. A straight leg raising deficit will almost certainly be noted but this is not specific for any one root.

762   Hydrocephalus means an increase in CSF volume within the skull. CSF is secreted by the choroid plexus, which passes out of the ventricular system through the foramina of the fourth ventricle, flows around the cerebellar and cerebral surface to be absorbed into the venous system through the arachnoid villi. A block of CSF flow at any point throughout its pathway or impaired reabsorption results in hydrocephalus. A block to flow may be caused by occlusion or narrowing of the foramen of Munro, the aqueduct of Sylvius or the fourth ventricle. This may result from tumour, congenital defect, haematoma or inflammatory exudate. Obstruction to reabsorption around the tentorial edge or at the arachnoid villi is usually caused by subarachnoid haemorrhage or meningitis. Rarely hydrocephalus is caused by excessive CSF secretion from a choroid plexus papilloma.

763   Patients with symptoms of raised intracranial pressure due to hydrocephalus require a shunt. Surgeons use ventriculo–atrial or ventriculo–peritoneal shunts depending on individual preference. These incorporate a valve system to prevent an excessive reduction in CSF pressure.

764   Harvey Cushing was a pioneer in neurosurgery working in Boston at the beginning of the century. He is recognized not only for descriptions of pituitary disease but also for his numerous advances in neurosurgical technique.

EAR, NOSE AND THROAT

765   Tympanometry is usually carried out automatically using a tympanometer. To obtain a tympanogram a probe from the tympanometer is inserted into the ear canal. This probe has three channels. One channel emits a sound and the

240

second channel is used to measure the amount of this sound reflected off the tympanic membrane. The third channel is connected to a pump which enables the air pressure in the ear canal to be varied. A tympanogram is a graphic representation of the way in which the amount of reflected sound varies in response to changing ear canal pressure. This can be used indirectly to measure middle ear pressure. For instance, in 'glue ear' the Eustachian tube is non-functioning and hence the middle ear space is poorly ventilated. The resulting low pressure fixes the tympanic membrane preventing it from moving in response to variations in ear canal pressure. As a result the amount of reflected sound will be constant and the tympanogram shows flat trace.

766 Prepare a clean aural syringe and about 200 ml of clean water at body temperature. Before proceeding, always ask the patient if he has had a perforated tympanic membrane or trouble resulting from syringing in the past — if in doubt do not proceed. Drape a towel over the patient's shoulder and ask him to hold a bowl to collect the water. Gently pulling the ear upwards and backwards with one hand, the nozzle of the syringe is just introduced into the external auditory canal with the other and the jet of water directed slightly upwards and forwards. When all the wax has been removed, the ear canal and tympanic membrane should be checked once more. If the procedure is painful or the wax shows no sign of moving, do not persist; instead refer the patient to an ENT surgeon. Complications resulting from incorrect aural syringing are a common cause of medicolegal complaints.

767 Malignant otitis externa is a Gram-negative infection in the external ear canal. It occurs classically in elderly diabetics. If untreated the infection spreads medially along the skull base and may cause cranial nerve palsies and death. Prolonged treatment is usually necessary with parenteral aminoglycoside antibiotics. Before the condition was fully recognized and understood, it had high mortality, hence the title 'malignant'.

768 If the discharge from the ear contains mucus, otitis media with a perforation is almost certainly present and characteristically, with an acute otitis

media, the pain disappears with the onset of discharge and there is no tenderness of the pinna or external auditory canal. In contrast, the purulent discharge of otitis externa is never mucoid and the pinna and external auditory canal may be very painful to the touch or on chewing. Deafness is an early feature in otitis media which frequently follows an upper respiratory tract infection, whereas deafness is not present, or is a late feature, in otitis externa. If the discharge can be cleared from the external auditory canal sufficiently to allow a view of the tympanic membrane, otitis media with a purulent discharge will always be associated with a perforation, in otitis externa the membrane is usually intact.

769 'Glue ear' (more correctly called secretory otitis media) is a condition in which fluid accumulates in the middle ear space because of a partial vacuum, the cause of which is a failure of the Eustachian tube to ventilate the middle ear adequately. This happens most frequently in children and commonly causes hearing loss. Eustachian tube malfunction occurs with adenoid hypertrophy, upper respiratory tract infections, nasal allergy and polyps, cleft palate, and tumours of the nasopharynx.

770 The organisms most frequently cultured in acute otitis media are *Streptococcus pneumoniae*, *Haemophilus influenzae*, beta-haemolytic *Streptococci* and *Staph. pyogenes*. *E. Coli*, *Proteus* and *Pseudomonas* are also encountered. Viruses probably also cause acute otitis media but they are difficult to identify.

771 The history is often characteristic. In safe (tubotympanic) chronic suppurative otitis media there are recurring episodes of mucoid or mucopurulent ear discharge, usually accompanying colds or 'flu, and associated with mild or moderate loss of hearing. In the unsafe (attico-antral) type there is often a history of constant and long-standing, foul smelling ear discharge associated with a more severe deafness. The distinction can usually be made for certain on otoscopic examination. In unsafe ear disease, there is a perforation of the tympanic membrane, either in the attic or posterior marginal region and cholesteatoma is often visible. In safe ear disease, the tympanic perfora-

tion is central and cholesteatoma is absent. Audiometry will usually confirm a more severe hearing loss in unsafe ear disease and plain X-rays and tomograms of the mastoids show sclerosis and sometimes bone erosion due to cholesteatoma. In safe ear disease, the mastoid is often pneumatized and there is no bone erosion.

772 The complications of long-standing, chronic, suppurative otitis media are due to erosion of bone and spread of disease to neighbouring structures. Erosion of bone by infection may lead to an extradural or subdural abscess. Extension superiorly gives rise to meningitis and temporal lobe abscess and posterior extension may cause thrombosis or septic thrombophlebitis of the lateral sinus, septicaemia or a cerebellar abscess. There may be paralysis of the 7th cranial nerve and erosion of bone medially leading to suppurative labyrinthitis and total loss of auditory and vestibular function. This may extend to involve the apex of the petrous temporal bone (petrositis) and lead to a 6th cranial nerve palsy and facial pain.

773 In otosclerosis, a focus of new bone formation encroaches upon the stapes footplate and prevents it from moving. The cause is unknown, although there is a variable genetic inheritance. Usually both ears are affected and it is thought that hormonal changes influence the new bone growth. For this reason women are affected more severely than men, especially if they have borne children. The deafness, which is conductive, starts early in adult life and is slowly progressive, although it never becomes total. So, in its classical form, otosclerosis presents as bilateral deafness in a young female with children, there is a family history of deafness and clinical examination of the ears reveals no abnormality apart from a pure conductive hearing loss.

774 The symptoms of Ménière's disease are deafness, tinnitus, vertigo and a feeling of pressure in the ear. One or both ears may be affected. The characteristic feature of the disease is the episodic nature of the symptoms — they may come and go in a marked and unpredictable fashion, but with an overall tendency towards deterioration over many years. The cause of the disease is not really under-

stood and no medical treatment has been shown to be curative.

775   An acoustic neuroma is a benign tumour of the supporting Schwann cell of the auditory (8th cranial) nerve. It usually presents with unilateral progressive sensorineural deafness and tinnitus. Occasionally there may be slight dizziness. When large enough to press on the brain stem and surrounding structures loss of balance may be more pronounced and there may be a partial 5th nerve palsy and symptoms resulting from raised intracranial pressure.

776   Although many patients with tinnitus have nothing seriously wrong with them, it is a common symptom and it may be very distressing. A search should always be made for a treatable cause. At the least, this means an examination of the ears and testing the hearing with a tuning fork and by pure tone audiometry. If the tinnitus is also audible to the examiner (so-called objective tinnitus) there is always a local cause, often of a vascular nature. Many common ear diseases, such as otitis media or otosclerosis, present with tinnitus and treatment may stand a good chance of bringing relief.

777   Presbyacusis means deafness due to ageing and is due to degenerative changes in the auditory pathway. Characteristically, the hearing is worse for high frequency sounds and this causes difficulty in hearing the consonants of speech. The result is that although the patient can hear that someone is speaking, he has difficulty in distinguishing the words. When a hearing aid is used, low frequency vowel sounds are often boosted to an uncomfortable level and this may make the use of a hearing aid unacceptable.

778   Whether or not a fracture can be demonstrated on a skull X-ray following head trauma, the presence of a CSF leak from the ear indicates that a fracture of the skull base is present. Prophylactic antibiotics should be given, for example Augmentyn or ciprofloxacin, because of the risk of meningitis. The patient should be nursed sitting up, if possible, to lower CSF pressure. A piece of sterile cotton wool can be placed in the external auditory meatus to soak up blood and CSF but otherwise

244

the ear should be left strictly alone. Usually, the CSF leak will stop spontaneously, but if it persists for more than 10 to 14 days a neurosurgical opinion should be sought to consider surgical closure of the dural tear.

779 Many broken noses are due to assault and careful records are important for possible medicolegal use later. The first step is to take a history and carry out a thorough examination to exclude other injuries, in particular associated fractures of the facial skeleton. If there are other injuries requiring urgent treatment, the nasal injury is of less immediate concern. First aid will usually control the epistaxis which follows a broken nose and lacerations are treated by toilet and suture as necessary. The septum should be checked for the presence of a haematoma (which requires early drainage, under general anaesthesia, if present) and X-rays of the nasal bones and facial skeleton should be taken. Bruising and swelling often prevent a full assessment of any deformity and the nose should be re-examined after 5 to 7 days. Significant displacement with cosmetic deformity will require manipulation within 14 days of the injury. If there is no visible displacement, manipulation is unnecessary.

780 The causes of nose bleeds are usually classified as local and general; the commonest local cause is exposed vessels in Little's area which are easily traumatised by children who pick at their noses. Repeated nose blowing because of colds often causes bleeding from the same region. Direct trauma to the nose, especially if a fracture is present, usually causes bleeding which stops spontaneously. Benign or malignant tumours in the nose are uncommon but may give rise to repeated minor epistaxes. Hereditary telangiectasia (Osler-Weber-Rendu disease) is also uncommon but almost always associated with nose bleeds. Of the general causes, systemic hypertension associated with atherosclerosis is far and away the most common. Diseases of the blood (factor and platelet deficiencies) also sometimes give rise to nose bleeds.

781 Treatment for nose bleeds is directed at correcting the underlying cause, such as hypertension, and arresting the haemorrhage. For minor nose

245

bleeds which arise from Little's area such as occur in children, first aid measures (sit up, lean forward, pinch the nose and breathe through the mouth) and sometimes cautery to the bleeding point with a silver nitrate stick are sufficient. For adults, especially when the bleeding point is posterior and inaccessible, some form of packing is often necessary — either anterior with ribbon gauze soaked in topical antiseptic (such as bismuth-iodine-paraffin paste) or posterior with a balloon catheter. Admission to hospital for bed rest, sedation and occasionally blood transfusion is then necessary. As a last resort, the maxillary or ethmoid artery may have to be ligated surgically.

782 Infections, particularly the common cold, invariably cause some degree of nasal obstruction. Vasomotor disturbance of the nasal mucosa, both allergic (hay fever) and non-allergic, are potent causes especially when vasoconstrictor sprays have been used repeatedly (rhinitis medicamentosa). Nasal polyps usually present with this symptom. Trauma may cause nasal obstruction which is reversible if due to mucosal swelling, but may be permanent if there is a deflection of the septum or organized septal haematoma. Large adenoids in young children and benign or malignant tumours in adults, and congenital choanal atresia complete the list.

783 Perennial allergic rhinitis is usually caused by dust or house dust mite and sometimes dietary factors. Steps to control or eliminate are recommended but on their own they are rarely sufficient. The mainstays of treatment are systemic antihistamines and topical nasal steroid sprays. Surgery to the turbinates (trimming, diathermy and cautery) may help to relieve nasal obstruction but rarely will do much for watery rhinorrhoea or sneezing fits.

784 This is an operation to correct septal deformity which may be congenital or traumatic. It entails elevating the nasal lining from both sides of the bony and cartilaginous septum and then removing or repositioning the deviated portion. The nasal lining is then allowed to come together in the midline and is usually held in place by a pressure pack in the nose for 24 hours.

246

785 Nasal allergy, which may be seasonal (hay fever) or perennial (for example dust allergy) is predominantly a Type 1 immediate hypersensitivity reaction mediated by IgE. The symptoms of nasal obstruction and discharge result from increased vessel permeability and oedema. This is caused by the release of histamine and other vaso-active substances from mast cells, as a result of the interaction between antigen and IgE.

786 In the strictest terms, sinusitis is an infection of the mucosal lining of the paranasal sinuses, whereas rhinitis (with which it is most often confused) is a vasomotor disturbance. Unfortunately, this distinction is often less clear cut in clinical practice because sinusitis may often cause rhinitis or vice versa. Classically sinusitis is associated with a purulent nasal discharge whereas the discharge of uncomplicated rhinitis is watery or clear and slimy. In both conditions, there may be facial pain, variable nasal obstruction and olfactory impairment. Sinusitis will usually be accompanied by abnormal X-rays whereas X-rays in uncomplicated rhinitis are often normal.

787 The treatment of sinusitis may be medical or surgical. Medical treatment entails identifying the causative organism with a nasal swab, aiding sinus drainage by the use of decongestant nose drops (such as Ephedrine), loosening secretions by the inhalation of steam and treating the infection with appropriate antibiotics. If an adequate trial of medical treatment fails to clear the infection, then an antral puncture and washout will often help by removing secretions and by obtaining a further specimen for culture. Formal surgical treatment is reserved for emergencies and failed medical treatment. Chronic maxillary sinusitis may be helped by making a large surgical opening for drainage into the nose (intranasal antrostomy). A similar drainage procedure is sometimes necessary for chronic infections in the frontal sinus. Acute infections of the frontal and ethmoid sinuses may lead to orbital cellulitis and a subperiosteal abscess requiring incision and drainage. In general, the advent of antibiotics has reduced the need to treat sinus infection surgically.

788   The paranasal sinuses are air spaces within bone. Most malignant tumours arise from the epithelium lining the sinuses and symptoms do not develop until the growth has filled the bony cavity and extended through the bone to involve neighbouring structures. This means that they present late, and usually only when local infiltration has taken place. The location of the nasal sinuses, close to the orbit and skull base, makes radical surgical removal difficult in many cases and unfortunately, the results of radiotherapy (the only real alterative to surgery) are equally poor.

789   Large tonsils and adenoids are the commonest cause of obstructive sleep apnoea in children. The size of the tonsils can easily be assessed by looking in the mouth. Adenoids are less easy to see on routine examination but can be well shown on a lateral X-ray. Oxygen saturation monitoring will confirm the diagnosis. Removal of the tonsils and adenoids is usually curative.

790   Traditionally the nasopharynx is examined with a bull's-eye lamp, head mirror, tongue depressor and warmed nasopharyngeal mirror. Special narrow diameter fibre-optic endoscopes are now available. These can easily be slipped through the nasal cavity a few minutes after the application of local anaesthetic/vasoconstrictor sprays to one or other nostril. Plain X-rays (a lateral of the skull and submentovertical view) give good imaging of the nasopharynx but where fine detail is needed CT or MRI are best.

791   Nearly half of all patients with nasopharyngeal cancer present with a symptomless lump in the neck as a result of cervical node metastases. If the Eustachian tube is obstructed, then there may be a complaint of deafness because of middle ear fluid. Facial pain and double vision result from direct upward extension into the skull base with involvement of the fifth and sixth cranial nerves. Nose bleeds may occur and be associated with nasal obstruction and 'catarrh'.

792   Aphthous ulcers are common and often occur on the lateral borders or undersurface of the tongue where they may be multiple. Trauma to the

tongue, whether accidental, or due to prominent teeth or an ill-fitting denture, may also lead to ulceration. Malignancy should always be suspected when an ulcer shows no sign of healing after 6 weeks and a biopsy is essential. Other causes of tongue ulcers include herpes virus infection and local manifestations of systemic diseases such as lichen planus, blood dyscrasia, Stevens-Johnson syndrome, vitamin deficiency and drug reaction (including Epanutin).

793 The Latin word globus means a sphere or ball and the term globus sensation is used to describe the common complaint of a feeling of a 'lump in the throat' usually at laryngeal level. The symptom is usually most noticeable between meals and may be relieved by eating. True difficulty in swallowing is absent. Although serious underlying disease is rare, a haemoglobin estimation and barium swallow should be carried out to exclude such conditions as the Patterson-Brown-Kelly syndrome, a pharyngeal pouch or carcinoma of the pharynx or upper oesophagus.

794 A pharyngeal pouch causes a rather vague difficulty in swallowing associated with regurgitation of food. When the pouch is large and laryngeal overspill has been occurring, there may also be repeated chest infections. Physical examination, including indirect laryngoscopy, rarely reveals anything. A barium swallow with AP and lateral views of the neck and thoracic inlet is diagnostic. Endoscopic examination will confirm the diagnosis but care must be taken because of the danger of perforating the wall of the pouch with the endoscope.

795 Post cricoid carcinoma is an epithelial malignancy arising from the hypopharyngeal mucosa where it lies against the posterior surface of the cricoid cartilage. It occurs predominantly in women and may complicate the Patterson-Brown-Kelly syndrome. The prognosis is poor (approximately 20% 5-year survival) especially if there are associated metastatic lymph nodes in the neck. This poor outlook, along with the often elderly and debilitated state of some of the patients, should be borne in mind when recommending treatment.

To achieve a cure radical surgery (pharyngo-laryngectomy) followed by radiotherapy probably offers the best hope. General measures to correct anaemia and improve nutritional status will usually be necessary pre-operatively. Surgery or radiotherapy alone may also be used for palliation when there is distressing dysphagia.

796   After 6 weeks at the latest. Although malignant disease of the larynx as a cause of hoarseness is uncommon by comparison with laryngitis or vocal abuse, early diagnosis is essential. Laryngoscopic examination is quick and easy to perform and the great majority of serious laryngeal diseases are visible. The cure rate for early cancers of the vocal cord is in the region of 90%, whereas the 5-year survival for advanced lesions, particularly if there are lymph node metastases, may be 25% at best.

797   In general a lesion obstructing the airway at laryngeal level will cause inspiratory stridor. If the lesion is in the trachea, the noise will be heard equally in inspiration and expiration, while airway obstruction below this level predominantly causes expiratory wheeze.

798   Epiglottitis is an infection of the epiglottis and supralaryngeal structures, usually occurring in children, with an acute onset and very rapid progression leading to severe airway obstruction. The time taken from onset to the development of stridor may be only a few hours and there is usually a high pyrexia and marked general malaise. *Haemophilus influenzae* is the most common organism responsible for the infection. Swabs and blood cultures should be taken and treatment consists of antibiotics (chloramphenicol is often used) and the relief of airway obstruction, either by tracheostomy or intubation. Steroids may be used to reduce inflammatory oedema.

799   The commonest causes of unilateral vocal cord paralysis are carcinoma of the bronchus involving the left recurrent laryngeal nerve, trauma during thyroid surgery and an idiopathic mononeuropathy. Other causes include bulbar palsy and carcinomas of the thyroid and oesophagus.

800 The treatment of laryngeal cancer is general and local. General measures include the correction of anaemia and nutritional deficiencies and treatment for chest infections. Local treatment may be curative or palliative. In the UK and Europe almost all laryngeal cancers are treated by radiotherapy in the first instance, to a maximum tolerated dose in an attempt to cure. Surgery is reserved for those patients who have received radiotherapy and in whom a biopsy has shown the presence of persistent or recurrent disease. Although removal of only part of the larynx is occasionally possible, surgery for most patients means a total laryngectomy. For those unfit for surgery or in whom only palliation is possible, chemotherapy or cryosurgery occasionally helps. If the tumour gives rise to airway obstruction a tracheostomy is sometimes necessary.

801 The first step is an attempt to make a diagnosis on the basis of the history and physical examination. With a lipoma or sebaceous cyst, this may be all that is necessary before proceeding to surgical removal if indicated. A lump apparently arising in the thyroid gland may require thyroid function tests or a scan before deciding on treatment. A problem arises when the lump has no special diagnostic features and when appropriate blood tests and X-rays have not helped with the diagnosis. A malignant lymph node is often suspected, in which case a thorough examination of the upper air and food passages should precede open biopsy.

802 The two main indications for tracheostomy are to allow prolonged artificial ventilation and to relieve airway obstruction. The former applies in major trauma and postoperative chest complications; if a peroral endotracheal tube cannot be removed after 10 to 14 days, tracheostomy is required to allow continued adequate tracheal suction and to reduce the dead space. Causes of acute airway obstruction include trauma to the head and neck as a result of traffic accidents, oedema due to allergy or infection and carcinoma of the larynx.

803 Close nursing observation and supervision are essential at all times during the first 24 hours after

a tracheostomy. This entails the provision of a special nurse or at least moving the patient to a bed adjacent to the nursing station. Humidification should be continuous for at least the first 3 days and suction should be carried out as often as necessary, but every hour at least. Without these precautions secretions become thick and viscous and dry to form crusts which obstruct the airway. Physiotherapy is necessary to help clear the chest since coughing is difficult when the larynx is by-passed. In addition, a sterile technique for dressings and the routine taking of swabs and sputum cultures will help identify any infections. The first tube change is done at around 3 to 5 days in the presence of a doctor.

THE EYES

804   There is either unilateral or bilateral proptosis associated with lid retraction and lid lag. Incomplete lid closure (lagophthalmos) may result in corneal drying due to interference with the blink reflex and exposure. Chronic inflammatory cell infiltration of the external ocular muscles may cause restricted eye movements and increased intra-orbital pressure. This in turn results in increased venous pressure, lid oedema and optic disc swelling. The two most serious complications which may lead to blindness are perforation of the eye due to exposure keratitis and optic nerve compression.

805   I would first measure the corrected distance visual acuities in each eye before testing the pupil reactions to light. I would then examine the anterior segment for evidence of inflammation (iritis) and both fundi, if possible through a dilated pupil. During this examination I would look for evidence of retinal or vitreous haemorrhage, a retinal tear or detachment, choroiditis or neoplasia.

806   The commonest cause of unilateral proptosis in a woman of this age is dysthyroid eye disease. Other less common causes include a meningioma, haemangioma, metastatic deposits from, for example, carcinoma of the breast or lymphoma.

252

807   Retinopathy of prematurity. This develops as a fibrovascular proliferation in response to excessive oxygenation of the immature retinal vasculature. The incidence may be reduced if the arterial Po_2 is monitored and should be maintained below 160 mmHg.

808   Blurring of vision due to papilloedema is a common presenting symptom of a cerebral tumour causing raised intracranial pressure. Involvement of the visual pathways by a tumour may produce gradually enlarging field defects and disorders of ocular movement may result from cranial nerve palsies. A ptosis or dilated pupil may be an early sign of a third nerve palsy and rarely tumours may present with a specific defect of accommodation. Finally, direct orbital extension of an intracranial tumour may cause proptosis.

809   Sarcoidosis may be manifested in the external eye by the presence of multiple small conjunctival granulomata or the presence of dry eyes due to lacrimal gland involvement. Anterior uveitis (iritis) is common and may be associated with the presence of iris nodules. Posterior segment changes include posterior uveitis, retinal vasculitis and optic disc swelling due to involvement of the optic nerve.

810   In conjunctivitis the inflammation is usually accompanied by a sticky mucous discharge and the pain takes the form of a gritty, foreign-body sensation. In iritis, pain is usually more severe with intense photophobia and may be accompanied by watering and blurred vision. The pattern of injection differs in the two conditions. In conjunctivitis it is said to be more inflamed towards the con-junctural fornices whereas in iritis, the inflammation is maximal around the cornea.

811   The ocular features include blepharitis, conjunctivitis, keratitis (which may be neuroparalytic in origin) and iritis with secondary glaucoma. Transient ocular motor palsies also occur sometimes. Ocular involvement in cases of herpes zoster ophthalmicus is said to be more common where the rash involves the side of the nose indicating involvement of the nasociliary branch.

812 A chalazion is a small hard nodule found in the eyelids which arises in the meibomian glands usually as a result of infection. Pathologically it has some of the features of a chronic granuloma and when it persists for more than a few weeks, it can be removed under local anaesthetic.

813 A dendritic ulcer is caused by herpes simplex virus infection of the cornea. Treatment consists of application of an antiviral ointment such as idoxuridine or acycloguanosine 5 times daily for up to 2 weeks or until healing has occurred. Photophobia may be relieved by a mydriatic or the wearing of dark glasses. Steroid preparations should never be used as these result in enlargement of the ulcer, delayed healing and increased scarring.

814 Fluorescein drops can be used to look for the presence of a corneal abrasion or ulcer. They can also be used to test the patency of the nasolacrimal duct. Injected fluorescein dye is used to perform fluorescein angiography in order to assess the retinal vessels and their associated pathology.

815 The diagnosis of a corneal abrasion would first be suspected from a history of trauma and confirmed by the instillation of fluorescein drops, which stain a corneal epithelial defect bright green. The treatment includes a mydriatic, e.g. atropine, to relieve pain as a result of ciliary spasm, antibiotic ointment, e.g. chloramphenicol, to prevent infection and a pad and bandage to keep the eye closed in order to encourage re-epithelialization. The eye should be inspected the following day in order to make sure that healing is occurring and that there is no infection.

816 Subconjunctival haemorrhage is most commonly idiopathic. Known causes include coughing, vascular abnormalities and blood dyscrasias. It may also occur following trauma and in these cases, if a posterior limit to the haemorrhage on the eyeball cannot be identified, bony injury to the orbit or anterior cranial fossa should be excluded.

817 The most important first aid measure is immediate irrigation using a cold tap or immersion in a bucket of cold water. In a casualty department,

the eye should be irrigated with buffered salt solution following local anaesthetic drops (amethocaine) — then the visual acuity assessed. Subsequent management depends on the precise nature of the chemical and if possible, a sample of it should be tested with universal indicator paper in order to discover its pH. Severe burns may require admission to hospital for intensive treatment with potassium ascorbate and steroid drops whereas minor burns (those not involving strong acid or alkali) may be treated with mydriatics and antibiotics.

818　Congenital melanin pigmentation of the conjunctiva is usually benign and of little significance. Acquired pigmentation however may indicate the development of a precancerous melanosis or a melanoma and therefore requires full investigation including biopsy.

819　An attack of acute glaucoma may start with the development of haloes (i.e. coloured rings around lights) associated with blurring of vision in one or both eyes. Later the eye may become painful and a severe headache develops. Nausea and vomiting may occur. The eye becomes congested with a vertically oval, fixed, semi-dilated pupil. The cornea is hazy and examination of the position of the iris shows a shallow anterior chamber. The eye feels hard, reflecting the increased intra-ocular pressure. The optic disc is difficult to visualize but it may be normal or swollen during an acute attack and may not appear atrophic until several weeks after the attack.

820　The most important complications are the formation of posterior subcapsular cataracts and the development of steroid-induced glaucoma. These can occur with prolonged topical or systemic therapy but are more common with the former. Topical steroid therapy will also adversely affect infective keratitis (particularly that due to herpes simplex virus).

821　This includes congenital abnormalities such as blockage of the lower end of the nasolacrimal duct, congenital entropion and trichiasis and congenital glaucoma (buphthalmos). Infective causes include ophthalmia neonatorum due to chlamydial infection.

822 Chronic simple glaucoma has an insidious onset and in its early stages the patient is usually asymptomatic. Later the patient may become aware of progressive defects in his visual field but these may not be noticed until the patient has tunnel vision as a result of gross peripheral field loss. Visual acuity is not reduced until a very advanced stage when the central fixation is affected. The cardinal sign of chronic simple glaucoma is the development of a pathologically cupped optic disc which is always associated with field defects.

823 Chloroquine and, to a much lesser extent, Hydrooxychloroquine produce corneal (cornea verticillata) and retinal toxicity changes (Bull's eye maculopathy). The latter does not reverse on withdrawal of the drug and if unrecognized will lead to blindness. Patients should have their eyes examined before starting treatment and monitored for any loss of the central red field by the use of a red Amsler chart.

824 Drugs may lower intra-ocular pressure by reducing aqueous secretion, promoting aqueous outflow or as osmotic agents. Acetazolamide is a carbonic anhydrase inhibitor which reduces aqueous secretion. Pilocarpine acts by constricting the pupil and pulling the iris root away from the trabecular meshwork, thus restoring the outflow facility to the eye. Intravenous mannitol or oral glycerol are examples of osmotic agents.

825 An intra-ocular foreign body should always be suspected where there is a history of metal striking metal at the time of an eye injury. The eye may look relatively normal if there is a small entry wound but the diagnosis is usually evident on examination of the pupil. A poorly reacting pupil suggests loss of the anterior chamber due to leakage of aqueous, while distortion of the pupil margin indicates iris prolapse or iridodialysis. If the fundal view through the pupil is obscured this may be due either to the presence of blood or to lens opacities. X-ray and/or ultrasound of the orbit should always be taken whenever the diagnosis is suspected.

826 Congenital cataracts may be associated with maternal infections such as rubella, cytomegalovirus

and toxoplasmosis. Other causes in children include Down's syndrome, Turner's syndrome, galactosaemia, Still's disease and severe atopic disease. In adults, the commonest condition associated with cataracts is diabetes mellitus but other less common associations include hypoparathyroidism and dystrophia myotonica. Steroids and chlorpromazine are examples of drugs which may induce cataract formation.

827 Pseudophakia is the term used to describe the presence of an artificial intra-ocular lens following cataract surgery. It is important because it allows the eye to continue to focus with a normal image size and thereby permits binocular vision where only one eye has been affected by cataract. It also avoids the need for cataract glasses which are unsatisfactory due to their magnifying properties.

828 Surgery may be indicated when bilateral cataracts prevent the patient from continuing normal activities; this usually occurs when the fully corrected visual acuity falls to approximately 6/18. Some patients require surgery at a much earlier stage, for example to maintain good driving vision or if they are troubled by glare. Occasionally surgery is required to improve visualization or treatment of retinal conditions, e.g. diabetic retinopathy.

829 The patient usually complains of discomfort behind the eye which is more marked on movement of the eye. The patient notices blurred vision due to the development of a central scotoma which may enlarge within hours, or more usually days to produce profound visual loss if fixation is affected.

830 There is a loss of the direct pupil reflex in the left eye with preservation of the consensual left response (when light is shone on the right eye). The pupil responses to accommodation are unaffected.

831 There is a pinkish discolouration of the disc associated with engorgement of veins and loss of spontaneous venous pulsation. Later the disc margins become blurred and the nerve fibres

swell to produce elevation of the disc. Gross papilloedema is associated with haemorrhages in the nerve fibre layer in and around the disc.

832   There are two main clinical types — background and proliferative retinopathy. Background retinopathy consists of the presence of microaneurysms, beading of veins, small blot haemorrhages and hard exudates. This form of retinopathy is associated with visual loss due to macular oedema or retinal capillary closure. Proliferative retinopathy is characterized by the formation of new vessels either in or on the retina or arising from the optic disc. Visual loss occurs as a result of haemorrhage into the vitreous or the development of fibrosis leading to secondary retinal detachment.

833   Yes. In background retinopathy, laser photocoagulation can be used to reduce macular oedema by coagulating leaking blood vessels. Early proliferative retinopathy is also treated with a laser but in advanced cases with retinal detachment the only treatment is surgical.

834   The patient may complain of blurred or distorted vision if the choroid near the macula is involved. A small focus of choroiditis may not produce any symptoms but floaters may develop due to the presence of inflammatory cells in the vitreous.

835   Choroidal melanoma commonly presents without symptoms as a pigmented lesion discovered on routine ophthalmoscopy. More advanced cases may present with secondary retinal detachment or secondary glaucoma. Distant metastatic disease (for example an enlarged liver), is a rare but well recognized form of presentation.

836   Night blindness is a defect in dark adaptation associated with abnormal function of retinal rods. It may be a congenital disorder not associated with any obvious fundus change, or it may be a presenting feature of inherited retinitis pigmentosa when the fundal changes include pigment clumping with narrowing of the retinal arteries and optic atrophy. The commonest cause of acquired night blindness is vitamin A deficiency when it may also be associated with keratomalacia.

837 Causes of sudden visual loss include retinal artery occlusion due to either embolism or thrombosis, central retinal vein or branch vein occlusion, vitreous haemorrhage, retinal detachment, optic neuritis and toxic optic neuropathy due to methyl alcohol poisoning.

838 Amblyopia is a condition of diminished vision which is not associated with any structural abnormality of the afferent visual pathways.

839 Pupil constriction occurs with parasympathetic stimulation either directly with acetylcholine and pilocarpine or indirectly with drugs which prevent the breakdown of acetylcholine such as physostigmine and phospholine iodide. Pupil dilatation is brought about either by sympathomimetic agents including adrenaline and phenylephrine or parasympathetic antagonists which include atropine, homatropine, hyosine and cyclopentolate.

840 There are three indications for squint surgery — to restore binocular single vision, to correct an abnormal head posture due to ocular torticollis and to produce a satisfactory cosmetic appearance.

841 Argon or Krypton lasers are used to photocoagulate retinal lesions e.g. diabetic retinopathy or subretinal neovascular membranes in age-related macular degeneration. Other forms of laser therapy include the use of YAG laser to create iridotomies in glaucoma or capsulotomies following cataract surgery. Recently eximer lasers have been used to treat corneal surface pathology and for the correction of refractive changes (e.g. myopia).

842 The differential diagnosis of a white pupil in childhood includes a congenital cataract, retinoblastoma, retinopathy of prematurity, choroiditis, retinal colobomata and persistent primary hyperplastic vitreous.

ORTHOPAEDICS AND FRACTURES

Fractures: general

843 The difference is that a compound fracture communicates with the exterior through a defect in

the skin, while a simple or 'closed' fracture does not. The importance lies in the danger of infection which is much greater in a compound fracture.

844 A pathological fracture is a fracture through bone which is abnormal for one reason or another. There are a large number of conditions which may weaken the bone, but a good example would be a secondary malignant deposit. Other common causes for pathological fractures are benign bone tumours (such as enchondroma) and Paget's disease.

845 A stress fracture is due to repetitive excessive loading on normal bone. A classic example is the march fracture in army recruits when fractures of the metatarsals are caused by a sudden increase in exercise stress. A more gradual increase in exercise should allow bones to adapt rather than fracture.

846 This is a common surgical emergency. The danger lies in the possibility that soft tissue or bony infection will occur. The patient should be given antibiotics and tetanus prophylaxis and then taken to theatre within 6 hours of injury. The wound should be surgically cleaned with removal of all contaminated or non-viable tissue, and in all but the most minor compound injuries the wound should be left unsutured. The fracture can be treated in various ways such as skeletal traction, internal or external fixation or plaster but, whichever is chosen, it should not interfere with dressing the soft tissue injury.

847 The principal danger is that swelling inside the rigid plaster will impair circulation to the distal part of the limb, resulting in gangrene. The danger can be avoided either by splitting the plaster until you can see the skin, or by initially applying a backslab and completing the plaster later.

848 Strong indications include failure of conservative methods, failure of reduction, an unstable fracture, a fracture involving a joint, and in multiple injuries. Other indications include delayed union or non-union.

849 An external fixator can be applied rapidly and provides speedy stabilization of fractures which is

particularly helpful in cases of multiple injury. It also has an important role when dealing with associated soft tissue injures. In this situation the bone is stabilized but access for dressings or skin grafting is maintained.

850   Callus is a mass of immature bone which forms as part of the healing process of a fracture. It forms a cuff around the broken bone ends and helps stabilize the fracture while union progresses. The callus is gradually remodelled to form mature bone but this process may take months if not years.

851   The standard classification is that proposed by Salter and Harris. Type 1 is through the growth plate, Type 2 includes a piece of metaphysis, Type 3 involves growth plate epiphysis, Type 4 involves epiphysis, growth plate and metaphysis and Type 5 is a crush injury of the epiphysis. The clinical importance is in the likely damage to the growth plate in Types 4 and 5.

852   This condition occurs following pelvic and long bone fractures and is characterized by a low Po_2 and consequent confusion leading on to unconsciousness if treatment is not instituted. There is widespread disturbance of gas exchange in the lungs. In some cases, a characteristic rash occurs on the upper half of the body.

853   The causes include excessive movement at the fracture site, distraction of the fracture, muscle interposition, sepsis, poor blood supply, synovial fluid in the fracture line, pre-existing bone pathology, advanced age, poor nutrition and steroid therapy.

854   In this condition there is a rise of pressure in one or more of the muscle compartments of a limb. This is often found following a fracture, although other types of injury may be responsible. When the pressure exceeds venous outflow pressure the veins collapse, leading to further increases in pressure and compartment muscle necrosis. The main clinical feature is severe pain. There is also paralysis, pain on passive stretching and sometimes paraesthesia. Frequently the distal circulation and pulses are normal. The main need is to diagnose the problem early. This is mainly ensured by a high index of suspicion, although

compartment pressure monitoring is helpful. An early thorough surgical decompression of all affected compartments is essential.

855 Nerve damage is divided according to its severity into three grades: neuropraxia, axonotmesis and neurotmesis. In neuropraxia conduction is interrupted for a short time only and will return fully in a matter of hours. Axonotmesis implies sufficient damage for axons to degenerate distal to the injury; however, the nerve is not completely disrupted and regeneration can be expected. In neurotmesis the nerve is completely disrupted and reinnervation will not occur without surgical repair. In practice these grades may co-exist in the same nerve, and give uneven recovery.

856 This is a childhood injury in which only one cortex of a bone is fractured. The bone may well be angulated and it may be difficult to correct the deformity without fracturing the remaining cortex. The bone has a tendency to spring back into the deformed position like a green stick. The immature skeleton will remodel deformities and the younger the child, the more remodelling will occur. Deformity is most commonly remodelled when fractures are close to the growth plate and the deformity is in the plane of movement of the adjacent joint. Rotational deformity is notorious for being unlikely to remodel with growth.

Orthopaedics: general

857 *Staph. aureus* is responsible in 80% of cases. It reaches the bone via the blood, usually from a septic focus elsewhere. The infection tends to lodge in the metaphyseal region of the bone where blood supply is greater.

858 The child is ill, pyrexial, anorexic, restless but not moving the affected limb which will probably be red, swollen, warm and is painful, particularly if moved. The white cell count and ESR are raised. The diagnosis can be particularly difficult to make in babies and should be borne in mind in the infant who is unwell with no obvious cause.

859 Acute osteomyelitis should be treated early and vigorously if compete resolution is to be achieved.

If chronic osteomyelitis is allowed to supervene then cure is extremely difficult to achieve. Blood cultures should be taken to try to identify the organism and high doses of bactericidal antibiotics should be given. Fucidic acid with flucloxacillin is a popular combination therapy. The place of surgery is not completely agreed upon but drainage should be performed if subperiosteal pus is thought to be present.

860   Dead bone, infected granulation tissue and pus within the bone, all part of chronic osteomyelitis, allow organisms to flourish, especially as penetration by antibiotics is poor in this condition.

861   Metal or cement predispose to bony infection and make eradication of infection more difficult. If an implant is inserted into a bone which has been infected in the past there is a considerable risk of making the infection active again.

862   The risk is about 1 to 2% of developing deep infection. To keep the rate as low as possible all septic foci should be treated before surgery. Prophylactic antibiotics have been shown to be effective and meticulous attention to sterility in the operating theatre is very important.

863   Rheumatoid arthritis, particularly when treated with steroids, presents some special hazards in surgery. Resistance to infection is lower, which is of particular importance when considering joint replacement. The bone is osteoporotic and will not hold surgical implants as well as normal bones. The skin is often thin and there may be a vasculitis leading to wound necrosis. Finally, it is important to X-ray the neck before embarking upon anaesthesia as there may well be a potentially unstable lesion in the cervical spine.

864   Débridement is the surgical cleaning of a wound including excision of all grossly contaminated, dead and doubtfully viable tissue. It is particularly important that dead muscle is carefully excised as it is a perfect culture medium for anaerobic bacilli.

865   The commonest deformity is an ulnar deviation at the MCP joints and it is very often accompanied by volar subluxation or dislocation of the

proximal phalanges on the metacarpal heads. The
joints may well be swollen due to the synovitis.
The mechanism of ulnar drift is not certain but
once it has begun the long flexor and extensor
tendons tend to increase the deformity.

866   Ankylosing spondylitis most commonly affects
young adult males. The spine and the costoverte-
bral joints are most commonly affected leading to
stiffness of the spine and poor chest expansion.
Later on, the spine may ankylose in a kyphotic
position leading to an ugly deformity. The large
joints, particularly the hips and knees may also
become progressively more stiff. Maintenance of
the range of movement and the use of anti-inflammatory drugs are the mainstay of treatment but
surgery can be useful. Joint replacement is often
very successful in these patients and in certain
circumstances spinal osteotomy may make a tre-
mendous difference to a severe kyphosis.

867   Osteoporosis is the loss of bone substance, including osteoid tissue, while osteomalacia is the
demineralization of bone without loss of osteoid.
Osteomalacia in children is known as rickets. The
blood chemistry is usually normal in osteoporosis
whereas in osteomalacia there is a high serum alkaline phosphatase and probably a high urinary
calcium.

868   Osteoporosis is a very common condition and is
always present to some degree in postmenopausal
females, making them more prone to fractures.
Disuse of the limb, due perhaps to immobilization in plaster, will cause osteoporosis while the
whole skeleton will be affected if a patient is confined to bed for a few weeks. Osteoporosis is an
accepted consequence of weightlessness experienced on a space flight. Rheumatoid arthritis and
the steroids that are commonly used to treat the
condition are both causes of osteoporosis.

869   Paget's disease of bone is a disorder of the normally continuous remodelling process. It may be
due to a virus but the aetiology is unclear. It is a
very common condition whose incidence increases with age, although it is usually asymptomatic. It causes the bones to become thicker and
to lose their normal internal architecture, so that
although they look widened and sclerotic on X-

ray, there is often bowing of long bones and pathological fractures may occur. When pain occurs it may be due to fissure fractures in the bowed and weakened bone. Secondary osteoarthritis may occur in adjacent joints. Two rare complications are high output cardiac failure due to bony arterial shunts and osteosarcoma which is rapidly fatal.

870 Achondroplasia is a failure of long bone growth due to poor ossification of cartilage. The long bones are more severely affected than the axial skeleton. An achondroplastic has short limbs, good musculature and normal intelligence. There is a risk of development of spinal stenosis and hydrocephalus.

871 Severe haemophiliacs are likely to get recurrent haemarthrosis of the major joints after little or no trauma; this can lead to severe secondary changes in the joints with fixed deformities. Such damage can be minimized by prompt splinting of the joint and treatment with factor VIII. Permanent damage to peripheral nerves can be caused by pressure from expanding haematomas and prompt measures are needed to prevent this.

872 Secondary deposits are far more common than primary bone tumours. Almost any tumour may spread to bone but there are five that classically do so — carcinoma of the breast, bronchus, kidney, thyroid and prostate. Simple clinical examination and investigation of these organs will often save the patient an unnecessary bone biopsy.

873 Osteosarcoma occurs most commonly in males between the ages of 10 and 30. The common sites, in order of frequency, are the lower end of the femur, upper tibia, upper humerus, distal radius and proximal femur. There are only 150 new cases of osteosarcomas a year in England and Wales and to detect such a tumour it is important to have an index of suspicion. Rarely, osteosarcoma is secondary to radiation therapy or Paget's disease.

874 It is important that investigation is performed in a centre accustomed to dealing with these rare conditions. The tumour is staged both locally and systemically by MRI, CT scanning as well as isotope

bone scan. The most likely sites for metastases are in the lungs and in bone. A biopsy is performed after the staging.

875 Osteotomy is surgical division and refixation of a bone. It may be used to correct deformities such as a bow leg; to reposition part of a joint, for example, the head of the femur in congenital dislocation of the hip; or for its non-specific pain relieving effect when a bone is divided near a joint.

876 Hemiarthroplasty is the reshaping or replacement of one half of a joint. The most common application is replacement of the head of the femur following subcapital femoral neck fracture in the elderly.

877 This depends a good deal on the weight and activity of the patient. It also depends upon the design of the prosthesis and the technique of implantation. An optimistic assessment would be 20 years for an active man aged 50.

878 The commonly used metals are stainless steel, chrome cobalt alloy, and titanium. A convex metal surface usually articulates with a concave surface of high density polyethylene. The other material in wide use is silastic, for the replacement of small joints such as in fingers and toes.

879 The most common problem is aseptic loosening of the joint which tends to occur some years after the original cause of failure. Other problems include recurrent dislocation and loosening due to infection.

Orthopaedics: regional

The hip and femur

880 True leg length is measured from the anterior superior iliac spine to the medial malleolus, while apparent length is measured from the umbilicus or xiphisternum to the medial malleolus. While true shortening indicates abnormality within the leg, apparent shortening is simply due to tilting of the pelvis. The most common cause of the tilting is a fixed adduction deformity at one hip which forces the patient to tilt the pelvis to avoid having to walk with his legs crossed.

881 The Trendelenburg is a test of the integrity of the abductor mechanism of the hip and is performed by asking the patient to stand on one leg. The test is positive if the opposite side of the pelvis drops down below the horizontal. The commonest cause of a positive test is pain due to arthritis in the hip, but it may also be positive if the abductor muscles themselves are weak or if the pivot around which they act is not functioning, for example after excision of the head of the femur. Trendelenburg also described a test for varicose veins.

882 Fixed flexion deformity of the hip is measured by the use of Thomas's test. In this test the patient lies on his back and any lumbar lordosis and pelvic tilting are eliminated by flexing the opposite hip as far as possible — a hand can be placed under the small of the patient's back to make sure the back is touching the couch. If the thigh comes off the couch there is fixed flexion deformity which is measured as the angle between the thigh and the horizontal.

883 The blood supply to the head of the femur runs in the capsule applied to the neck of the femur with little if any supply via the ligamentum teres. The vascularity of the head is therefore endangered if the capsule is stretched or disrupted. This may occur with fracture of the neck of the femur, dislocation of the hip joint or the maintenance of an extreme position of the hip joint as may occur during treatment for congenital dislocation of the hip.

884 The bony contours of the ball and socket articulation provide considerable stability, enhanced by the fibrocartilagenous labrum around the edge of the acetabulum which deepens it. The thick joint capsule, condensed to form the iliofemoral, pubofemoral and ischiofemoral ligaments, and the muscles which cross the hip joint add to the stability. Considerable force is required to dislocate this joint.

885 Typically this fracture produces a shortened, externally rotated, painful leg. In the elderly, who are particularly susceptible to this fracture, and in the demented, pain may not be severe and inability to walk may be more important as a clinical

feature. If the fracture is impacted, the classical deformity will not be present and the patient, although complaining of pain, may be able to walk. Therefore an X-ray is necessary in the elderly patient complaining of hip pain. The mortality approaches 30% by 3 months, primarily due to the loss of mobility in an elderly patient leading to pneumonia, bed sores, urinary infection, deep vein thrombosis etc.

886   Replacement of the femoral head following *intracapsular* fracture is the usual treatment because the alternative, reduction and pinning, has drawbacks in this injury. These include the likelihood of non-union of the fracture, avascular necrosis of the head of the femur, and cutting out of the pin from osteoporotic bone on attempted weight bearing. Replacement of the head of the femur, although a more major procedure, allows early return to full mobility, so vital in the elderly patient.

887   Posterior dislocation of the hip requires considerable violence and may therefore be associated with other severe injuries which may distract attention from the hip. The most likely decoy is an ipsilateral fracture of the femoral shaft which will account for pain in the region and will disguise the characteristic fixed adducted posture which the dislocated hip will assume. Posterior dislocation of the hip joint should not be missed if a careful examination of the patient is undertaken.

888   Central dislocation of the hip is really a fracture-dislocation in which the head of the femur is forced through the acetabulum into the pelvis. The head of the femur is itself quite likely to have received considerable damage. Reconstruction is very difficult and a good result unlikely.

889   This condition should be diagnosed as soon after birth as possible as treatment is then easier and more effective. It is a clinical diagnosis, reached during routine examination of the infant. The main clinical signs are loss of abduction and a clunk or click of reduction which occurs when the hip is placed in the stable position of flexion and abduction. Asymmetry of skin creases may be seen around the hip joint in a unilateral disloca-

tion but this is an unreliable sign. Later on there is development of a fixed flexion deformity and further limitation of abduction. Radiology is not of much help until the proximal femoral epiphysis begins to ossify at the age of 3 or 4 months.

890   If congenital dislocation of the hip is treated early it is usually quite easy to obtain a sound reduction, and from there development of the hip proceeds normally. On the other hand, if the dislocation is not discovered until the child has learned to walk, a number of secondary deformities are likely to have developed, making treatment considerably more difficult — open reduction of the dislocation may then be required and osteotomies of the femur and pelvis may be needed to obtain a stable hip.

891   The condition is commoner in females by a factor of six. The other risk factors are breech presentation, first-born babies, oligohydramnios, Caucasian race and positive family history. It is important to know the epidemiological facts about CDH so that those at risk may be carefully watched.

892   The pathological process in Perthes' disease is one of recurrent episodes of avascular necrosis of the whole or part of the femoral capital epiphysis, the cause of which has not been established. If the degree of necrosis is minor, then replacement of the dead bone occurs without permanent disability, while if a large amount of the head is affected, collapse of the femoral head will occur with varying degrees of flattening when healing finally occurs.

893   The most common difficulty is due to tightness of the adductor muscles. This leads to limited abduction and eventually to subluxation or dislocation of the hips. Such problems can often be prevented by regular physiotherapy.

894   A mild or moderate pain in the groin or knee may be the only symptom. The patient, usually a young adolescent, may develop a slight limp and later a deformity consisting of shortening and external rotation of the affected leg. This is a deceptive condition and may be difficult to diagnose.

895 A lateral X-ray of the hip is needed because the slip tends to occur in a posterior direction and may be missed in the early stages if only an AP film is taken. Adequate hip X-rays may not be ordered if the patient's pain is mainly in the knee.

896 The common causes include Caisson's disease (diver's and tunneller's occupational hazard), alcohol ingestion, steroid treatment and Cushing's disease and sickle-cell disease. There is also a group of patients in whom the cause is not known.

897 The presence of sepsis elsewhere in the body is an important contra-indication which must be dealt with before operation is performed. Old sepsis around the affected joint is also a considerable danger. Loss of bone stock for any reason means that it is very difficult to fix the components of the hip joint securely to the bone. Youth is a relative contra-indication to total hip replacement as revision operations are more likely to be required in the younger and more vigorous patient.

898 An acute septic arthritis of the hip should not be difficult to diagnose except in a very young child unable to indicate the site of pain. The hip is stiff and painful to move and there is a severe systemic upset with pyrexia and a raised white cell count and sedimentation rate. Less acute infection may be more difficult to identify particularly in a deep joint such as the hip. In such cases, aspiration of the hip, as well as the usual blood cultures, may be necessary to establish the diagnosis.

899 In the early stages there is some joint space narrowing, particularly superiorly. Later bony sclerosis develops while subchondral cysts and osteophytes form around the joint.

900 The femur should be splinted, an intravenous infusion started, blood taken for cross-matching, and analgesia given. Splintage, usually with a Thomas's splint, will minimize further damage to soft tissues, reduce bleeding into the thigh and lessen pain. Volume replacement should be started early as blood loss into the thigh may be up to 2 litres. Analgesia should be given before all the painful steps associated with radiological examination, provided there are no contra-indica-

tions such as head injury. Small intravenous doses of opiate are preferable to intramuscular injections which may be absorbed very slowly in such circumstances. In short, emergency treatment aims to stabilize the general condition prior to definitive treatment of the fracture.

901 At the scene of the injury the femur should be immobilized with any available splint or even by bandaging to the uninjured limb. Modern inflatable splints are easier to apply than the Thomas splint. Once the patient arrives at the hospital it is preferable to undertake definitive fixation within the first 24 hours. This will usually be in the form of a locked intramedullary nail.

The knee and lower leg

902 The menisci perform two useful functions — they act to spread a considerable proportion of the load across the knee joint so that point loading does not occur, and they have a role in spreading synovial fluid around the joint and thus nourishing the articular cartilage. The menisci used to be thought to have little if any use, so that their removal would do little damage. However, it has now been shown that their removal causes considerable damage to the joint and is likely to lead to osteo-arthritis of the knee.

903 In adults there is a physiological valgus of about 7° between femur and tibia. There is a range of normality between about 2° and 11° with women tending towards the higher values. In children these angles do not apply as very small children often develop bow legs followed by knock knees and end up perfectly normal adults. The physiological valgus must be taken into account in total knee replacement.

904 A 'locked' knee has a block to full extension, usually as a result of trauma. This may be quite a subtle sign, with only the last few degrees of normal hyperextension missing from the range. Sometimes intermittent locking will occur, when the patient finds the knee will not straighten past a certain point; however, if he manipulates the knee, suddenly the full range of movement returns. The usual causes of a locked knee are a torn meniscus or a loose body in the knee.

905 Lateral or medial strain should be applied to the knee in about 20° of flexion, as the anatomy of the knee is such that it is stable to such strains when fully extended, even if the collateral ligaments are divided. It is important to test the other knee as the degree of normal laxity varies considerably from person to person. Isolated collateral ligament damage is rare — the cruciate ligaments and possibly other structures may have been injured as well.

906 If the knee is damaged for any reason there is rapid wasting of the quadriceps muscle. The vastus medialis is the component that shows this wasting first and is usually the last to recover. Other muscles in the limb will undergo wasting but the quadriceps is particularly important as it contributes to the strength and stability of the knee. Rehabilitation programmes for the knee are designed primarily to rebuild quadriceps power.

907 It may be difficult to do this acutely because of pain and it may be necessary to repeat the examination later or perform it under anaesthesia. The classic test is 'anterior draw' when the knee is bent to 90° and, with the foot immobilized, the examiner checks the degree of forward subluxation of the tibia against the uninjured knee. A more physiological test is Lachman's test when the anterior draw is tested in 25° of flexion instead of 90°.

908 Plain films of the knee are essential and it may well be useful to take a condylar view and a skyline view of the patella to look for osteochondral injuries. Valgus and varus stress views may also be useful. The arthrogram has now largely been superseded by the MRI scan which is very useful indeed in a wide variety of knee injuries.

909 Tears most commonly begin in the posterior region of the medial meniscus. This area of the meniscus can be caught between the femur and tibia by a sudden twist on the flexed knee. Once the tear has begun it is likely to extend round to the front of the meniscus and may eventually produce a complete 'bucket handle' tear.

910 It used to be thought that removal of the meniscus was a harmless procedure, but on long-term

follow up it has been shown that osteo-arthritis of the knee is a common consequence which may occur many years later. It has also become apparent from autopsy studies that asymptomatic meniscal tears are common; for this reason surgeons are becoming more conservative in their indications for meniscectomy.

911 Aspiration of the knee will help to relieve pain and will also provide diagnostic information. Blood in the joint indicates a substantial injury and any fat globules suggest a fracture has occurred.

912 This is a condition in which there is gradual separation of an osteochondral fragment from a surface within the knee joint. The commonest site is on the lateral side of the medial femoral condyle. It often occurs in athletic teenagers and young adults, causing pain and swelling with occasional locking or giving way, particularly if the fragment becomes completely separated.

913 Unstable patella is a term which describes a range of conditions. In its mildest form this can be a slight abnormality of tracking of the patella in the intercondylar groove leading to retropatellar pain. At the opposite end of the scale is congenital dislocation of the patella when the patella lies lateral to the knee joint. Between these extremes the patella may subluxate or dislocate with varying degrees of readiness. The mildest degrees of instability may be helped by physiotherapy aimed at increasing muscle control of the patella but in more marked instability some form of surgical realignment of the patella is required.

914 Genu varum is bow legs. In this condition the weight of the body is taken mainly or entirely through the medial compartment of the knee joint, leading to loss of articular cartilage. In advanced cases there may be bony collapse of the medial tibial plateau or the medial femoral condyle which will make the deformity worse. Pain is caused by the degenerative arthritis on the medial side of the joint and possibly also by traction on the lateral ligamentous structures.

915 This operation is most commonly performed to correct varus deformity of the knee associated with osteo-arthritis confined to the medial com-

partment of the knee. With increasing success of total knee replacement, the indications for osteotomy are less frequent but it is still the operation of choice in the younger patient with this condition. The operation is performed for other deformities but the results are not as good or as predictable as for the varus deformity.

916 A displaced fracture needs accurate repair or possibly excision of the patella and repair of the expansion, after which the knee is splinted for some weeks. If a fracture is undisplaced, the extensor mechanism remains intact, so that splintage is necessary only for a short period.

917 In Osgood-Schlatter's disease the patellar tendon pulls on the apophysis of the tibial tubercle and produces gradual avulsion with new bone formation. This is due to disproportion between the strength of the quadriceps and the hardness of the bone. As the apophysis closes the symptoms will resolve.

918. It should be at least 13 cm from the knee to allow a suction fit prosthesis. The stump should have a well healed and mobile scar with sound skin. It is important that there is good soft tissue cover and that the nerve ends are well away from the end of the stump so as to avoid tender neuromata.

The ankle and foot

919 Arthrodesis of the ankle will give a pain free result. Although there is loss of movement, there is still some dorsi/plantar flexion available at the mid-tarsal region. Ankle arthroplasty is not suitable for osteo-arthritis although there is a limited place for the procedure in a polyarthritis.

920 Sprained ankle is usually an inversion injury with damage to the lateral ligament of the ankle joint, the anterior and middle components of this ligament usually receiving the brunt of the damage. In the majority of cases there is only a partial tear and full recovery occurs, but if there is a complete tear of one or more of the components of the lateral ligament there may be a permanent disability.

921 In ankle fractures the final functional result is closely correlated with the accuracy of reduction. Large forces pass through this complex joint which has a relatively small surface area so that any small malalignment or roughness of the surface leads to wear of the articular cartilage.

922 A bunion is a bony exostosis, often covered by a bursa, which produces a bump on the medial aspect of the head of the first metatarsal bone. Hallux valgus means angulation of the big toe in a lateral direction, leaving the head of the first metatarsal more obvious than usual. A bunion often accompanies hallux valgus, making the symptoms worse.

923 Hallux rigidus is osteo-arthritis of the first metatarsophalangeal joint. There is gradual onset of stiffness and pain and the formation of bony osteophytes around the joint, particularly on the dorsal aspect. The condition may follow old trauma or unusual strains such as occur in sporting or dancing activities.

924 Metatarsalgia is pain in the forefoot due to excessive weight bearing on one or more of the metatarsal heads, in turn producing a callosity under the foot which makes the painful area more prominent. There are several causes including toe deformities, such as claw toe; previous surgery for hallux valgus, which may stop the big toe functioning as a weight-bearing organ; fixed plantar flexion at the ankle; and loss of soft tissue padding from the sole of the foot, as may occur in rheumatoid arthritis.

925 The other name for club-foot is talipes equino varus. This term provides a description of the deformity — 'equinus' refers to plantar flexion of the foot and ankle as occurs naturally in the horse (equus), and varus refers to inversion of the foot. In severe club-foot there is a tight tendo Achilles and a high, small, inverted heel and some adduction of the forefoot. The calf and foot are smaller than normal, this becoming more noticeable as the patient gets older and persisting even if a good correction of the deformity has been achieved.

926 Flat feet are common in the young and do not cause symptoms in this age group. Later in life, as muscles and ligaments weaken, there may be further collapse of the longitudinal arch and symptoms may develop. Some flat feet may have a marked valgus deformity which may be painful. The most troublesome form of flat foot, requiring early treatment, is the rocker-bottomed foot, due to a congenitally vertical talus — in this condition the sole is actually convex and the position of the talus can be seen on X-ray.

The spine

927 An AP, lateral and odontoid (open mouth) view. It is very important to ensure that the full extent of the cervical spine is seen on the film and it may be difficult to show the C7/T1 region. Oblique and flexion/extension views may also be helpful and an axillary of 'swimmers' view' may help to show the C7/T1 region.

928 This has made an enormous difference to the investigation of the spine. It has almost eliminated the need for invasive investigations such as radiculography and discography. It is excellent for demonstrating all space-occupying lesions in the spinal canal, as well as bony abnormalities.

929 An intervertebral disc consists of an outer layer of concentric rings of tough fibrous tissue known as the annulus fibrosis and a semi-fluid interior called the nucleus pulposus. The fibres of the annulus lie at 45° to the vertebrae and alternate layers are at right angles to each other. The nucleus pulposus, the remnant of embryonic notochord, is situated towards the posterior part of the disc. This structure allows mobility as well as efficient shock absorption.

930 Structural scoliosis, that is, a fixed rotation of the vertebrae, can best be seen if the suspected area is viewed in profile and is accentuated when the patient bends forward, when the ribs will emphasize the deformity. Another clue may be given by a high shoulder or prominent hip.

931 Limitation of straight leg raising by pain indicates tethering of the lower lumbar nerve roots, usually

due to a prolapsed intervertebral disc. A useful confirmatory sign of this pathology is the sciatic stretch test, in which the leg is raised to the level that pain permits and the foot then passively dorsiflexed — this will cause pain due to further traction on the nerve roots. Both legs may have limited straight leg raising due to tight hamstrings but this is not painful.

932   A patient with spondylolisthesis of significant degree has a shortened lumbar region with a fold in each flank and a loss of normal lordotic curve. A step may be palpable in the lumbar spine.

933   The most reliable method is to fit a skull halo and a jacket which will allow the patient to mobilize while keeping the neck safely immobilized. Other methods include cervical collars which lack the stability offered by the halo.

934   A psoas abscess will point in the groin as it tracks down the psoas tendon. The other important sign is hip flexion due to psoas spasm.

935   This is a condition that usually occurs in later life. The patient describes pain and numbness and deadness in both legs. This occurs with exercise, particularly when walking uphill and it is rapidly relieved by sitting down. It is important to distinguish this condition from vascular claudication.

936   This disabling condition can be prevented much more effectively than it can be treated. It is important to identify those at risk and offer them hormone supplementation and advise regular exercise. Calcium supplements and diphosphonates have a much more limited effect.

937   In the lower cervical spine. This area, which is prone to injury, is often poorly shown on X-ray due to lack of co-operation in a patient who may be drunk or concussed. By pulling down on the arms or by taking oblique views it is possible to show this area in sufficient detail to exclude injury.

938   The vast majority of prolapsed intervertebral discs will resolve with conservative management. The patient should be rested in bed with adequate nursing and analgesia until symptoms have sub-

sided. He can then be mobilized slowly and advised on the avoidance of back pain. Some patients will benefit from physiotherapy and weight loss. Only a small percentage of disc prolapses require surgery.

939   A disc that prolapses in a directly posterior direction, so that the sacral nerve roots are damaged bilaterally, is an urgent matter requiring early treatment. Interference with bladder function is a sign that this has occurred and early decompression is necessary. If decompression is delayed there may be permanent urinary incontinence.

940   The term 'laminectomy' is often used loosely to mean the same as 'disc excision'. Laminectomy means removal of the lamina of a vertebra so that the spinal canal is completely decompressed; this approach was once used for disc excision but it is now reserved for more extensive operations inside the spinal canal. Disc excision is usually carried out through a more limited exposure in which the ligamentum flavum is removed with only a small portion of the adjacent lamina.

941   Spondylolisthesis means the slippage of one vertebral body forwards on the one below, usually at the L5/S1 or L4/5 levels. Spondylolysis is a break in the pars interarticularis and is one of the causes of a spondylolisthesis. Spondylosis means osteoarthritic changes of the spine and is the most common of these three conditions.

942   Posterolateral fusion, possibly combined with root decompression, is the most common surgical procedure. Some surgeons advocate a more radical approach in which the deformity is reduced after a major soft tissue release followed by fusion in the reduced position. However, spondylolisthesis need not be treated unless the slip is progressing or it is causing pain.

943   The most common type of scoliosis is the adolescent idiopathic type. This condition usually affects girls and produces a progressive curve, convex to the right, in the thoracic region. It is a particular problem because it can develop rapidly, producing an ugly rib hump at an age when girls are particularly sensitive about their appearance.

944 The patient should be nursed flat on pillows and rolled regularly on to his side. The pelvis and thorax are moved as one so that no twisting strain is put on the damaged area. Various special beds are available which make regular turning easier.

945 In rheumatoid arthritis the neck may be unstable, leading to cord injuries during intubation and anaesthesia. In particular atlanto-axial subluxation can occur leading to cord transection by the odontoid process. Therefore careful pre-operative assessment is essential.

946 An unstable injury of the cervical spine should be reduced and then the reduction maintained. Reduction is usually obtained and held by skull traction. A halo-jacket apparatus may later be substituted to permit mobilization. Sometimes internal fixation is used.

947 If patients recovered from the shock of the original injury they soon became affected by chronic urinary infection, contractures of the affected limbs and by pressure sores. The death of such patients was often extremely unpleasant, associated with infection from sores or from urine. If breathing was affected by the injury, then pneumonia was another major cause of death.

The shoulder and arm

948 The arm is held abducted and appears longer than the opposite side. The rounded outline of the shoulder disappears because the humeral head is displaced and instead there is a sharper angulation caused by the prominent acromion. There is a fullness of the subcoracoid region where the humeral head comes to rest. Movement is not possible at the shoulder in an acute dislocation.

949 Approximately one-third of total shoulder movement occurs at the scapulothoracic articulation and the remaining two-thirds at the glenohumeral joint. This means that even after arthrodesis of the glenohumeral joint there is still a useful range of movement at the shoulder.

950 The rotator cuff is composed of the tendons of supraspinatus, infraspinatus, subscapularis and teres minor muscles. They blend with the capsule of the shoulder joint and act primarily as stabilizers of the humerus on the glenoid to allow other muscles such as deltoid and pectoralis major to work effectively. The rotator cuff muscles can act as prime movers, particularly in the early stages of abduction, but their main function is one of providing stability.

951 The circumflex nerve arises from the posterior cord of the brachial plexus. It leaves the axilla via the quadrilateral space (between teres major, subscapularis, the long head of biceps and the surgical neck of the humerus). It gives a branch to the shoulder joint and then divides into deep and superficial branches. The deep branch runs round the neck of the humerus and penetrates deltoid to supply it. A small patch of skin over the tip of the shoulder has sensory supply from this nerve. The superficial branch supplies teres minor and then becomes superficial at the posterior border of deltoid and becomes the upper lateral cutaneous nerve of the arm.

952 If the lateral view of a shoulder is unclear it is useful to have an axial view, in which the X-ray tube is placed in the axilla and a plate exposed on the superior aspect. This will show the humeral head articulating with the glenoid and can rule out dislocation. If the shoulder is very painful a film can still be obtained without abduction of the arm being necessary. The patient is simply tilted back 20° and a satisfactory picture can be obtained without causing pain.

953 At a cursory examination, the shoulder is not obviously abnormal in posterior dislocation as the displaced head is concealed as compared with its prominence in anterior dislocation. In addition, this dislocation commonly occurs following electrocution or epilepsy so that the patient is unlikely to be in a fit state to complain of pain in his shoulder. Furthermore, a plain PA X-ray may not show the dislocation while a lateral may well be unsatisfactory because of overlying shadows of the thorax — an axial view is needed.

954 Reduction of a dislocated shoulder should be as gentle as possible to avoid further damage to soft tissues. In a fresh injury this should be easy, but after a few days the soft tissues become tight and open reduction may be required. In the acute case some patients will spontaneously reduce if they are laid prone with the injured arm dangling over the side of the bed. Most require manipulation under sedation or under general anaesthesia and muscle relaxation. The two popular methods of manipulation are Kocher's manoeuvre and the Hippocratic method. In Kocher's manoeuvre the surgeon applies traction in lateral rotation and 30° of abduction. The limb is then adducted and internally rotated simultaneously and this should obtain reduction. In the Hippocratic method the surgeon pulls on the arm and with his stockinged foot guides the head of the humerus into position. This method does not consist of yanking as hard as possible against the counter-pressure of the surgeon's foot in the armpit. If reduction is not achieved by closed methods there is no shame in resorting to open reduction which is a great deal safer than repeated forceful closed manipulation.

955 Recurrent dislocation of the shoulder is usually secondary to an initial traumatic dislocation. In the original injury the anterior capsule of the shoulder was injured and the glenoid labrum torn away from the bone leaving a defect, the so-called Bankart lesion. This sharp edge of glenoid can make a dent in the humeral head which is known as a Hill-Sachs lesion. In external rotation and abduction the shoulder is likely to slip out of joint if these lesions are present. Surgical repair consists of an anterior approach to the shoulder and a procedure to tighten up the capsule and repair the Bankart lesion.

956 Usually this is a trivial fracture which will heal if supported in a triangular sling and if mobilization is allowed as soon as pain permits. The other common method of treatment is a figure-of-eight bandage to hold the shoulders back and so, hopefully, to reduce deformity. This is an uncomfortable treatment and is only necessary if cosmesis is particularly important to the patient. Open reduction and internal fixation are very rarely indicated.

957 Although this fracture is generally thought of as being trivial it must be remembered that a number of vital structures can be injured. The great vessels of the root of the neck, the brachial plexus and the trachea can all be damaged. Sir Robert Peel fell off his horse and a sharp fragment of clavicle lacerated the subclavian vein. He died from loss of blood.

958 Totally different principles of treatment are involved in the two types of sling. A collar-and-cuff sling supports the arm from the wrist, applying traction to the upper arm and is therefore used for fractures of the humeral shaft. Conversely, a long arm sling supports the arm under the elbow and so would cause angulation of a humeral shaft fracture, but it is useful to rest an injured shoulder, a fractured clavicle or a subluxed acromioclavicular joint.

959 'Frozen shoulder' is an adhesive capsulitis of the shoulder joint. There is thickening and fibrosis of the joint and the capacity of the capsule is markedly reduced so that there is restriction of movement in all directions. It may be post-traumatic but in other cases the aetiology is unclear.

960 In this condition, a segment of the arc of abduction is painful, while the rest of the arc is pain free. It is caused by a degenerate or inflamed area of the supraspinatus tendon being squeezed between the humeral head and the acromion during this segment of abduction.

961 The rotator cuff consists of a hood of the conjoined tendons of subscapularis, supraspinatus and infraspinatus muscles. This band of tendons holds the humeral head into the glenoid and stabilizes the shoulder allowing the other muscles to act around a stable fulcrum. A tear of the rotator cuff prevents effective abduction of the shoulder.

962 Colles' fracture occurs most commonly in the elderly female and is usually caused by a fall on the outstretched hand. There is a fracture of the distal radius with shortening, dorsal displacement and angulation — the dinner fork deformity. Often there is an associated fracture of the ulnar styloid.

963 The aim of treatment in Colles' fracture in the elderly is to preserve movement and function — restoration of exact alignment is a secondary aim. If there is more than 20 to 30° of dorsal angulation, the fracture is manipulated under local or general anaesthesia and reduction is held with a plaster back slab reaching from the upper forearm to the metacarpal necks. The manipulation consists of disimpaction by traction, exaggeration of the deformity to align the dorsal cortices and then volar and ulnar manipulation. The plaster should hold the wrist in moderate palmar flexion and ulnar deviation with pronation of the forearm. Swelling of the fingers is prevented by elevation in a high sling for a few days and by encouraging early use of the fingers, elbow and shoulder. The plaster is completed once swelling is subsiding and X-rays should be taken at 1 and 2 weeks after the injury to check that the reduction is maintained. At about 6 weeks after injury, the fracture will have united and mobilization out of plaster can begin.

964 A Monteggia fracture-dislocation is a fracture of the upper third of the ulna with dislocation of the radial head. Sometimes the radial head dislocation is missed as the X-ray may not quite include the whole length of the bone. It is unusual for only one bone in the forearm to be fractured so that damage to the proximal or distal joints must be carefully excluded.

965 This fracture is well known for producing the disastrous complication of Volkmann's ischaemic contracture. The brachial artery can quite easily become occluded or divided, so very careful observation is needed to detect ischaemia early. If it is detected, operation to decompress the artery and the fascial compartments must be performed immediately.

The hand

966 The deep flexor tendons act on the terminal phalanges of the digits and function is tested by active flexion of the terminal interphalangeal joint while the examiner immobilizes the rest of the finger. The superficial flexor tendons insert into the

middle phalanges and are tested by asking the patient to flex one finger at a time while the others are kept straight by the examiner, a manoeuvre which eliminates the mass action of the deep flexor.

967   The median nerve supplies the radial side of the palm of the hand, the palmar surface of the radial three and a half digits and the dorsal aspect of their terminal phalanges. The ulnar nerve supplies the ulnar one and a half digits and the ulnar side of the hand on both the dorsal and palmar aspects. The radial nerve supplies the dorsal aspect of the radial side of the hand and the proximal part of the dorsal aspect of the radial three and a half digits. There is considerable variation in the sensory innervation and also a good deal of overlap which may become apparent if one nerve is injured.

968   The skin becomes dry and warm and feels smooth to the touch. Dirt does not stick to dry skin as easily as moist skin and this may show up the denervated area on the radial side of the hand. There is wasting of the thenar eminence and loss of power of abduction of the thumb. Provided the nerve injury is a low one there will be no impairment of the long flexors but pinch grip is likely to be affected.

969   The hand lies in a characteristic posture of clawing of the little and ring fingers due to paralysis of the intrinsic muscles. The hand is markedly wasted, especially the hypothenar eminence and on the dorsal aspect between the metacarpal bones. There is loss of abduction and adduction of all the fingers but the intrinsic muscles most easily tested are the first dorsal interosseous muscle which normally abducts the index finger and abductor digiti minimi which abducts the little finger. There is sensory loss over the ulnar side of the hand and the ulnar one and a half digits.

970   Abductor pollicis brevis is innervated by the median nerve in at least 99% of subjects. It is tested by laying the hand on a flat surface with the palm up. The patient is asked to lift the thumb straight up away from the palm and this power is tested against resistance.

284

971 The main deficit is loss of finger and wrist extensor function. It is difficult to open the hand enough to grasp large objects, but the power of grip is also weakened. The sensory deficit on the back of the arm and hand is not usually a major problem.

972 There are four main types of grip — the power grip, in which all the fingers close round the gripped object; the chuck grip, involving the thumb, index and middle fingers and which gives fine control of movements as when holding a pen; the pinch grip, between the pulp of the index finger and thumb; and the key grip, between the tip of the thumb and the radial side of the index finger.

973 The blood supply of the scaphoid can only enter via a strip of bone on the dorsal aspect of the waist of the bone as a large proportion of its surface is covered in articular cartilage. A fracture across the waist of the scaphoid incurs a considerable risk of avascular necrosis of the proximal fragment of bone.

974 In trigger finger there is a tendency for the finger to become stuck in full flexion. It can be extended either by active effort or by passive extension when it becomes free with a snap. The long flexor tendons catch in the fibrous flexor sheaths at the level of the distal palmar crease which may be due to tightness of the sheath, thickening of the tendon, or proliferation of local synovium, the cause of which is usually unknown.

975 Elevation of the limb is an effective way of minimizing oedema and is best achieved by using a roller towel at the side of the bed. If a sling is worn the hand must be kept high. Movement is very important in pumping away oedema fluid and so preventing stiffness, so early movement should be encouraged. Infection is a very potent cause of stiffness and drainage of any infection and treatment with antibiotics should be particularly vigorous in the hand.

976 Total loss of either power or sensation in the hand is a serious disability but loss of sensation is particularly crippling. The affected hand is liable to

repeated injury and infection. Provided the arm is able to place a paralysed hand it can still perform an important function if sensation is normal.

977　This injury, which occurs most commonly in young men, causes localized pain and tenderness over the anatomical snuff box. Most fractures are undisplaced and often not detectable on the X-ray taken shortly after the injury. If strongly suspected clinically, treatment should be started even if X-rays are normal — this consists of immobilization in plaster from the forearm to the metacarpal heads including the thumb. Repeat X-rays at 10 days, including oblique views, will usually demonstrate the fracture if present. Healing takes from 8–12 weeks on average but non-union and avascular necrosis of the proximal pole sometimes occur, when operative treatment needs to be considered.

978　Most such fractures can be treated by splintage to the adjacent finger and encouraging early movement. Stable fractures must be differentiated from the unstable for which other forms of treatment are required.

979　Bennett's fracture is really a fracture-dislocation of the base of the thumb. A blow on the metacarpal causes a fracture through the base of the bone extending into the joint. Usually a small triangular piece of bone is left in its normal place and the rest of the bone is subluxated or dislocated laterally.

980　The area known as 'no-man's land' is between the distal palmar crease and the middle phalanx of the digit. In this area the deep and superficial flexor tendons lie within a fibrous sheath and are very likely to form adhesions. For this reason orthodox teaching was that no man should perform a primary repair of flexor tendons in this region.

981　This is in the middle of no-man's land and primary repair can easily lead to severe adhesions. Primary repair is acceptable treatment, but only if it is performed under the best possible conditions. In other words the wound should be fresh and caused by a sharp instrument with no crushing or gross contamination of tissue. In addition the surgeon should be experienced in tendon surgery

286

and have the right equipment to perform it. If there is doubt on any of these scores it is better to go for early wound healing and mobilization of the finger, and a secondary tendon graft at a later date.

982 Infections are more damaging in the hand than elsewhere because they quickly lead to swelling and stiffness. Fibrosis around a focus of infection, while causing little functional effect in most parts of the body, may profoundly upset the function of the hand.

983 Treatment of pus in the hand should be vigorous and early — this includes both drainage of pus and full antibiotic therapy. The hand should be elevated and mobilized early to reduce oedema and to prevent stiffness.

984 This is an avulsion of the extensor tendon from the base of the distal phalanx. A common mechanism is a blow on the end of the finger as may occur in football or cricket. It is usually treated conservatively in an extension splint for 6 weeks.

985 A grease-gun injury occurs when lubricant is accidentally injected into the hand under pressure and requires early and vigorous treatment. The injected material spreads in the tissue planes and may end up a long way from the injection site producing a lot of swelling and fibrosis. Treatment consists of early surgical excision of all injected material. Other industrial materials such as oil or paint may be involved in this type of injury.

986 This injury almost always occurs from punching someone in the mouth. The cut may be small but is very likely to be highly contaminated and there is often a piece of tooth embedded in the wound. It is important to treat this injury seriously and perform a complete surgical débridement and to give full doses of antibiotics. The metacarpophalangeal joint is likely to be involved and sepsis here will produce a very awkward stiff finger.

987 Usually the patient first notices pain and tingling in the radial three and a half digits although it often includes the whole hand and may spread up the arm as far as the shoulder. The symptoms tend to be worse at night, often wakening the pa-

tient, and may be relieved by hanging the arm over the side of the bed. If symptoms persist, motor changes are likely to occur with wasting of the thenar eminence and weakness of abductor pollicis brevis. The patient often complains of a tendency to drop things.

988   De Quervain's Syndrome comprises pain over the tendon sheaths of flexor pollicis brevis and abductor pollicis longus with palpable thickening. It is due to stenosing tenovaginitis of the tendon sheaths at the radial styloid. It may be helped by local injection of steroids but surgical release is usually required.

989   Dupuytren's disease occurs most commonly in men aged over 40, sometimes in association with chronic liver disease. It usually starts with thickened nodules of fibrous tissue in the palms of the hands and this extends into the little and ring fingers to cause progressive contractures of the metacarpophalangeal and proximal interphalangeal joints. Progression is usually very gradual but in some patients, particularly the younger ones, it can be more aggressive and cause multiple severe contractures. There are frequently pads of tissue on the dorsal aspect of the finger joints and nodules of Dupuytren's tissue are sometimes found on the soles of the feet.

990   A ganglion is a cyst arising from a synovial cavity, either a joint or a tendon sheath, usually about the wrist. They are smooth and fluctuant and contain clear, glary fluid. They are often asymptomatic but if they give trouble they can be excised although there is a chance of recurrence.

WHAT IS . . . ?

991   A cyst is a collection of fluid in a sac lined by epithelium or endothelium. The word originates from the Greek work for bladder.

992   A fistula is an abnormal track connecting two epithelial surfaces.

993   A sinus is a blind track leading away from an epithelial surface into surrounding tissues, and lined by granulation tissue.

994 An ulcer is a defect in an epithelial surface due to progressive cellular destruction rather than sudden trauma.

995 A carbuncle is an area of subcutaneous gangrene, due to staphylococcal infection. The lesion most commonly occurs at the back of the neck.

996 An empyema is a collection of pus in the pleural cavity. The term is also used for an abscess in an obstructed hollow viscus, particularly the gallbladder or appendix.

997 This is a development abnormality of lymphatics and consists of a mass of lymphatic cysts. It is usually found in the neck, jaw or axilla and is brilliantly transilluminable.

998 In a case of obstructive jaundice, if the gall-bladder is palpable, then the jaundice is not due to stones in the common bile duct.

999 Sister Marie-Joseph's nodule is a secondary deposit seen in the umbilicus in cases of intra-abdominal malignancy.

1000 *Editors' comment:* Throwing an obscure name at you is a ploy beloved of examiners. If Gazornenplat wasn't the middle European inventor of a variety of pyloroplasty, jejunostomy or herniorrhaphy, then beware — having noted your Alma Mater, the examiner may be inviting you to hang yourself by showing total ignorance of the name of your recently retired Professor of Surgery, a phenomenon all too common amongst generations of medical students!